Aging in Cell and Tissue Culture

Aging in Cell and Tissue Culture

Proceedings of a symposium on "Aging in Cell and Tissue Culture" held at the annual meeting of the European Tissue Culture Society at the Castle of Žinkovy in Czechoslovakia, May 7-10, 1969

Edited by

Emma Holečková
Institute of Physiology
Czechoslovak Academy of Sciences
Prague, Czechoslovakia

and

Vincent J. Cristofalo
Associate Member
Wistar Institute of Anatomy and Biology
Philadelphia, Pennsylvania

PLENUM PRESS • NEW YORK–LONDON • 1970

Library of Congress Catalog Card Number 70-110800

SBN 306-30470-8

© 1970 Plenum Press, New York
A Division of Plenum Publishing Corporation
227 West 17th Street, New York, N. Y. 10011

United Kingdom edition published by Plenum Press, London
A Division of Plenum Publishing Company, Ltd.
Donington House, 30 Norfolk Street, London W.C. 2, England

FOREWORD

The annual meeting of the European Tissue Culture
Society was held at the Castle of Žinkovy in Czechoslovakia
from May 7-10, 1969. Included as part of this meeting was
a symposium on "Aging in Cell and Tissue Culture." This
volume contains the papers presented at that symposium.

The use of cell and tissue culture techniques to
study the mechanism of aging is not new. For example,
it has long been known that age-associated changes which
occur in plasma can inhibit cell proliferation in vitro;
also that the time lapse prior to cell migration from explanted tissue fragments increases with increasing age.
These are both examples of the expression in vitro of
aging in vivo. More recently, attention has been focused
on the occurrence of senescence in vitro. These investigations have included studies of alterations in non-
dividing cell cultures, and to a somewhat greater extent,
of age-related changes in the proliferative capacity of
cells in vitro. For example, cells derived from human
fetal lung retain many properties of normal cells including
a stable normal diploid karyotype and these cultures have
been shown to have a limited life-span in vitro. In addition, cultures derived from human adult lung show the same
normal characteristics and appear to have a shorter lifespan than cells derived from fetal lung.

The gerontologist, of course, is interested in whether aging in vitro bears any relationship whatsoever to aging in vivo and whether studies carried out in tissue culture have any relevance to aging in the whole animal. On the basis of the evidence now available, the strongest support for the relevance of studies with proliferating cell cultures to aging in vivo lies in, first, the well-documented age-related increases in the latent period of tissue explants, and second, the reports that cell cultures derived from adult tissue have a significantly shorter life span than those derived from fetal tissue.

Added support for this position might be provided by the results from several more controversial areas of investigation. For example, there is the question of the species specificity of the limited life-span of normal cells; if the phenomenon is truly relevant to aging in vivo, then it should be a characteristic for cultures taken from all vertebrate species. Human and avian cells in vitro seem to follow the general rule that normal cells have a limited life-span; however, there have been several reports of rodent cells which maintain their proliferative capacity for what appears to be indefinite periods, without any major variation in karyotype. One must realize, of course, that the karyotype represents only one of the the criteria applied to normal human cells.

A second area of controversy concerns whether the observed senescence in vitro is truly dependent on an intrinsic programmed function of the cell or is due to nutritional deficiencies or the trauma of cultivation.

A third as yet unresolved question is whether the decline
in the proliferative capacity of the cells really depends
on the number of cell generations rather than on the time
the cells have spent in culture, that is, the "metabolic
lifetime" of the cells.

This symposium brings together people whose work
can shed light on some aspects of these questions. The
major emphasis of the symposium is upon studies of the
capacity for cell proliferation after aging in vivo
(latent-period studies) and during aging in vitro. Dr.
Hay reviews his work and that of others with cell lines
derived from a variety of species. He places in perspec-
tive the various lines of evidence bearing on the question of the species specificity of the limited lifetime
in vitro of normal cells, on the environmental versus
the senescence basis for this limited life-span, and on
the question of whether in vitro aging is dependent on
time-related changes or on cell doublings.

The presentation of Dr. Soukupová and her colleagues
carefully documents the fact that there is an increase in
the latent period of a number of rodent tissues with age
after the animal reaches maturity. Dr. Macieira-Coelho
provides further support for the correlation between aging
in vivo and in vitro. He demonstrates that human fibroblasts of adult origin, during the first part of their
life in vitro, show patterns of division that are
characteristic of human fibroblasts of embryonic origin
which are entering the final stages of their lifetime in
vitro.

Dr. Simons points out in his presentation that to
establish the relevance of cell culture studies to aging
in vivo, a correlation of some kind must be demonstrated
between comparable studies in vivo and in vitro. In his
work with cultures derived from _Potorous tridactylis_, a
marsupial with six pairs of easily recognizable chromosomes, he found that cultures of embryonic heart cells
express symptoms of senescence very similar to those in
cultures of human fetal lung cells. In addition, he has
shown that cell volume and its variability are directly
correlated with aging.

In their presentations, Drs. Kritchevsky and Howard,
Cristofalo, and Michl and Svobodová all describe data concerned with the changes in various biochemical parameters
associated with cell aging in culture. These include age-
associated increases in the cellular content of lipids
and RNA, a decrease in the stability of RNA during aging,
and the variability of the activity of certain enzymes
during aging.

Dr. Stanek's description of time-lapse cinemato-
graphy of the death of individual cells in vitro suggests
that the death of cells in culture under certain conditions may be a purely individual event and completely unrelated to the death of any other cell in that culture.

The speakers at this meeting have defined many
of the problems connected with aging at the cellular
level. Very little is really known about the process of
aging in vivo. Certainly it must be a complex phenomenon

involving various mechanisms and different kinds of cells
and tissues. The aging of neurons probably proceeds by
a different mechanism than that of the continually proliferating tissues, such as skin and blood-forming elements. Macromolecules, such as collagen and elastin, represent a third component with their own mechanisms of
senescent degeneration. Then there is the effect of interaction among these components and the resulting senescent changes that ensue. Thus, it is very difficult
with the present state of our knowledge to pinpoint the
relationship between cell proliferation in vitro and aging
in vivo; however, it would seem, in the light of current
evidence, that these age-associated changes in proliferative capacity represent a very useful model for the aging
of at least some types of tissues and quite possibly represent the aging of these components at the less complex
cellular level. This concept has provided a new tool for
the science of gerontology and in studies, which are now
really just beginning, application of this concept has
given rise to new and exciting approaches to our understanding of the problems of aging and death.

This is the first time that papers presented in
conjunction with the annual symposium of the European
Tissue Culture Society have been published. The symposium brought together the ideas and results of scientists from varied backgrounds and disciplines, from both
the United States and Europe, all of whom are interested in the use of tissue culture techniques to
study aging. We hope that the publication of this
volume will reflect the value of the exchange of in-

formation and ideas which occurred at Žinkovy Castle and which is so important to this relatively new approach to gerontological research.

We regret the absence of printed discussions. At the time of the meeting, however, we were not certain that the proceedings would be published and so no record was made of the interesting and lively discussions which occurred.

We would like to extend our thanks to Dr. David Kritchevsky of the Wistar Institute for his help in planning the publication of this volume; to the Plenum Press for its efforts in making rapid publication of this volume possible; and to Mrs. Lucinda Rose of the Wistar Institute for her editorial services in preparing this manuscript. The editors are grateful to the Czechoslovak Academy of Sciences for its support of the meeting; funds for this publication were provided, in part, by U.S. Public Health Service Research Grant RO1-HD 02721 from the National Institute of Child Health & Human Development.

Emma Holečková
Institute of Physiology
Czechoslovak Academy
of Sciences
Prague, Czechoslovakia

Vincent J. Cristofalo
Wistar Institute of Anatomy
and Biology
Philadelphia, Pennsylvania

LIST OF PARTICIPANTS

M. ALBRECHT, Städt. Krankenhaus Moabit, Turmstrasse 21,
1 Berlin 21, Germany.

E.J. AMBROSE, The Chester Beatty Research Institute,
Fulham Road, London S.W.3., England.

G. ASTALDI, The Blood Research Foundation Center,
Municipal Hospital, Tortona, Italy.

O. BABUŠÍKOVÁ, Research Institute of Oncology, Ul.čsl.
armády 17, Bratislava, Czechoslovakia.

V. BAJOVÁ, Department of Infectious Diseases of the
Veterinary Faculty of Medicine, Komenského 71,
Košice, Czechoslovakia.

K. BANKOVÁ, Institute of Pathological Anatomy, Hněvotínská
3, Olomouc, Czechoslovakia.

G. BARSKI, Institut Gustave-Roussy, Centre Clinique et
Thérapeutique, 16 Bis Av. Paul-Vaillant-Couturier,
94 Villejuif, France.

U. BATZDORF, University of California, Department of
Surgery, School of Medicine, The Center for Health
Sciences, Los Angeles, California 90024, U.S.A.

M. BAUDYŠOVÁ, Czechoslovak Academy of Sciences, Institute
of Physiology, Budějovická 1083, Praha - Krč,
Czechoslovakia.

S. CARPENTIER, Institut de Progénèse, Université de Paris,
15, rue de l'École de Médecine, Poste 293, Paris 6e,
France.

Z. CHOLVADTOVÁ, Department of Plant Physiology, Komenský
   University, Odborárske nám.12, Bratislava,
   Czechoslovakia.

O. CINNEROVÁ, Czechoslovak Academy of Sciences,
   Institute of Physiology., Budějovická 1083, Praha -
   Krč, Czechoslovakia.

V. CRISTOFALO, The Wistar Institute, Thirty-sixth Street
   at Spruce, Philadelphia, Pa. 19104, U.S.A.

Z. DEYL, Czechoslovak Academy of Sciences, Institute of
   Physiology, Budějovická 1083, Praha - Krč,
   Czechoslovakia.

V. DRASTICHOVÁ, The Clinic of Plastic Surgery, Berkova
   34, Brno - Královo Pole, Czechoslovakia.

D.M. EASTY, The Chester Beatty Research Institute, Fulham
   Road, London S.W.3., England.

J. FEIT, Institute of Pathological Anatomy, Medical
   Faculty, J.E. Purkyně University, Pekařská 53, Brno,
   Czechoslovakia.

A. FERLE-VIDOVIĆ, Institute "Ruder Bošković", Bijenicka
   54, Zagreb, Yugoslavia.

H. FIRKET, Institut de Pathologie, Laboratoires d'Anatomie
   Pathologique, 1 Rue des Bonnes-Villes, Liège, Belgium.

L.M. FRANKS, Tissue and Organ Culture Unit, Imperial Cancer Research Fund, Lincoln's Inn Fields, London W.C.2.
   England.

J. GAYER, Institute of Biology, Faculty of Medicine,
   Charles University, Šimkova 870, Hradec Králové,
   Czechoslovakia.

A. GROPP, Pathologisches Institut der Universität Bonn,
   Gewebezüchtungslaboratorium, Bonn/Rhein, Venusberg,
   Germany.

O. GROSS, Institut d'Histologie et d'Embryologie, 9 Rue
du Bugnon, 1000 Lausanne, Switzerland.

B. GRZELAKOWSKA-SZTABERT, Department of Biochemistry,
Tissue Culture Laboratory, Nencki Institute of Experimental Biology, Pasteura 3, Warsaw 22, Poland.

W. HALLE, Institut für Kreislaufforschung der DAdW,
Lindenberger Weg 70, 1115 Berlin-Buch, Germany,(DDR).

A. HAMANN, Universitäts-Frauenklinik, Homburg-Saar,
Germany.

W. HAMANN, Pathologisches Institut der Universität,
Albertstr. 19, 78 Freiburg, Germany.

R. HAY, Department of Embryology, Carnegie Institute,
115 W. University Parkway, Baltimore, Md. 21210, U.S.A.

S. HÉBERT, Institut d'Histochimie Médicale, 45 Rue des
Saints-Pères, Paris VI, France.

P. HNĚVKOVSKÝ, Biological Institute, Faculty of Medicine,
Charles University, Albertov 4, Praha 2, Czechoslovakia.

E. HOLEČKOVÁ, Czechoslovak Academy of Sciences, Institute
of Physiology, Budějovická 1083, Praha - Krč,
Czechoslovakia.

F. KALAFUT, Research Institute of Oncology, Ul.čsl. armády
17, Bratislava, Czechoslovakia.

V. KESZEGHOVÁ, Research Institute of Oncology, Ul.čsl.
armády 17, Bratislava, Czechoslovakia.

J. KIELER, Fibiger Laboratoriet, Lundtoftevej 5, Kongens
Lyngby, Denmark.

H. KOBLITZ, Institut für Faserstoff-Forschung der DAdW,
153 Teltow-Seehof, Berlin, Germany (DDR).

P. KOŘINKOVÁ, Czechoslovak Academy of Sciences, Institute
of Physiology, Budějovická 1083, Praha - Krč,
Czechoslovakia.

J. KOZIOROWSKA, Department of Tissue Culture and Viro-
    logy, Serum and Vaccine Research Laboratories, 30-34
    Chelmska str., Warsaw, Poland.

D. KRITCHEVKSY, The Wistar Institute, Thirty-sixth Street
    at Spruce, Philadelphia, Pa. 19104, U.S.A.

H. LETTRÉ, Institut für Experimentelle Krebsforschung der
    Universität Heidelberg, Vossstrasse 3, Heidelberg,
    Germany.

R. LETTRÉ, Institut für Experimentelle Krebsforschung der
    Universität Heidelberg, Vossstrasse 3, Heidelberg,
    Germany.

H. LIMBURG, Universitäts-Frauenklinik, Homburg-Saar,
    Germany.

D.R. LUCAS, Medical Research Council, Radiobiological
    Unit, Harwell, Didcot, Berkshire, England.

A. MACIEIRA-COELHO, Institut de Cancérologie et Immuno-
    génétique, 14, Av. Paul Vaillant Couturier, 94
    Villejuif, France.

T. MAGROT, Institute of Biology, Faculty of Medicine,
    Charles University, Karlovarská 48, Plzeň,Czechoslo-
    vakia.

J. MICHL, Czechoslovak Academy of Sciences, Institute of
    Physiology, Budějovická 1083, Praha - Krč,
    Czechoslovakia.

E. MITROVÁ, Institute of Histology and Embryology, Faculty
    of Medicine, Komenský University, Sasinkova 1,
    Bratislava, Czechoslovakia.

L. MORASCA, Instituto di Richerche Farmacologiche, "Mario
    Negri" 20157 Milano, Via Eritrea 62, Italy.

S. MOSKALEWSKI, Department of Histology, Medical Academy,
    Chalubinskiego 5, Warsaw, Poland.

J. MOTAJOVÁ, Slovak Academy of Sciences, Institute of
Virology, Mlýnská Dolina, Bratislava, Czechoslovakia.

D.G. MURPHY, Adult Development and Aging Branch, National
Institute of Child Health and Human Development,
National Institutes of Health, Bethesda, Maryland
20014, U.S.A.

M.R. MURRAY, College of Physicians and Surgeons, Columbia
University, 630 West 168th Street, New York, N.Y.,
U.S.A.

E. MÜLLER, Institut für Biochemie der Pflanzen der DAdW
zu Berlin, Weinberg, Halle/Saale, Germany (DDR).

D. PETROVIĆ, Institute "Ruder Boškovič", Bijenička 54,
Zagreb, Yugoslavia.

D. PETRŽELKOVÁ, Czechoslovak Academy of Sciences, Laboratory of Otolaryngology, U nemocnice 2, Praha 2,
Czechoslovakia.

M. POSPÍŠIL, Czechoslovak Academy of Sciences, Institute
of Microbiology, Department of Immunology, Budějovická 1083, Praha - Krč, Czechoslovakia.

V. PÖSSNEROVA, 1. Clinic of Internal Diseases, U nemocnice 2, Praha 2, Czechoslovakia.

D. ŘEZÁČOVÁ, Research Institute of Immunology, Šrobárova
48, Praha 10, Czechoslovakia.

A. SCHABERG, Pathologisch-Anatomisch Laboratorium,
Wassenaarseweg 62, Leiden, The Netherlands.

J.P. SCHERFT, Laboratorium voor Celbiologie en Histologie, p/a Rijnsburgerweg 10, Leiden, The Netherlands.

A. SCHLEICH, Institut für Experimentelle Krebsforschung
der Universität Heidelberg, Vossstrasse 3, Heidelberg, Germany.

B. SEKLA, Institute of Biology, Faculty of Medicine,
   Charles University, Albertov 4, Praha 2, Czechoslovakia.

J.W. SIMONS, Department of Radiation Genetics,
   Wassenaarseweg 62, Leiden, The Netherlands.

J. SKŘIVANOVÁ, Institute of Biology, Faculty of Medicine,
   Charles University, Albertov 4, Praha 2, Czechoslovakia.

M. SOUKUPOVÁ, Institute of Biology, Faculty of Medicine,
   Charles University, Albertov 4, Praha 2, Czechoslovakia.

V. SPURNÁ, Czechoslovak Academy of Sciences, Institute
   of Biophysics, Královopolská 135, Brno 12,
   Czechoslovakia.

H. STÄHELIN, Sandoz, AG, 4000 Basel, Switzerland.

I. STANEK, Institute of Histology and Embryology, Faculty
   of Medicine, Komenský University, Sasinkova 1,
   Bratislava, Czechoslovakia.

M. STÁREK, Research Institute of Immunology, Šrobárova
   48, Praha 10, Czechoslovakia.

J. SVOBODA, Czechoslovak Academy of Sciences, Institute
   of Experimental Biology and Genetics, Flemingovo 2,
   Praha 6, Czechoslovakia.

J. SVOBODOVÁ, Research Institute for the Medical Use of
   Radioisotopes, Budějovická 800, Praha - Krč,
   Czechoslovakia.

L. ŠEFČOVIČOVÁ, Research Institute of Epidemiology and
   Microbiology, Sasinkova 9, Bratislava, Czechoslovakia.

S. TANNEBERGER, Robert-Rössle-Klinik der DAdW, Lindenberger
   Weg 70, 1115 Berlin, Germany (DDR).

I. TÖRŐ, Department of Histology and Embryology,
    Tuzeltò-u.58, Budapest IX, Hungary.

S. TRANEKJER, Universitäts-Frauenklinik, Homburg-Saar,
    Germany.

J. UHER, Postgraduate Medical and Pharmaceutical Insti-
    tute, Praha - Podolí, Czechoslovakia.

C.M.J. VERNE, Institut d'Histochimie Médicale, 45 Rue
    des Saints-Pères, Paris VI, France.

M. VRBA, Research Institute of Pediatrics, Černopolní 9,
    Brno, Czechoslovakia.

R. WIDMAIER, Institut für Experimentelle Krebsforschung
    der DAdW, Lindenberger Weg 70, 1115 Berlin-Buch,
    Germany (DDR).

CONTENTS

xix

*   *   *

OPENING REMARKS

At the annual meeting of the European Tissue
Culture Society in Davos in 1967, Professor Gaillard
proposed that symposia on topics that are ripe for
discussion should be included in the regular program
of the meetings.

It is probably not rash for me to say that there
are several areas in biology and medicine in which
tissue culture methods have not only contributed a
great deal to our insight into fundamental biological
problems but also have revealed new phenomena and
offered new approaches to their study and understanding.

In 1968, in London, Dr. Barski introduced the first
of these symposia on hybridization of somatic cells in
culture. Participants in that symposium had an opportunity to follow the intricate events of cell and
nuclear fusion and to admire both the quantity of data
available and the elegance of the methodology which had

been developed for the study of hybrid cells in the short
time since the exciting discovery of somatic cell matings.

This year the second symposium, on aging in cell and
tissue culture, brings a very old but recently revived
problem into focus. The study of aging in tissue culture
(or by tissue culture methodology) is practically as old
as the technique of tissue culture itself. The finding
that it is usually much easier to obtain actively proliferating explants from embryonic tissues than from tissues of older donors was made by Carrel and his co-workers
as early as 1910*. Since that time every student of tissue culture has sooner or later rediscovered this fact.
The positive correlation between the length of the latent
or lag period of explanted tissues and the chronological
age of its donor has been widely known for half a century,
but the reasons for this correlation remain obscure. In
primary tissue explants, the extracellular substances and
the body fluids, to the extent that they reflected ontogenetic changes, were accused of being at least partly
responsible for the observed decrease of cellular migration and mitosis in vitro. Much has been learned about
the nature of these changes which occur with age in both
these kinds of substances (which are, of course, products
of specialized cell types in vivo), and, as is usually
the case in science, much more remains to be learned.
Nevertheless, these practical approaches have achieved a
certain amount of success, elucidating, for example, some
of the changes which occur with age in collagen molecules
or the effects of various serum protein fractions upon
cellular growth in vitro.

*A. Carrel and M.T. Burrows, J. Am. Med. Assn., 55:1379,
  1910.

The history of aging in tissue culture also has its
philosophical side. Everyone is probably aware of the
idealistic concept that death is the price which the
organism has to pay for its high degree of organization, while the happy anarchy of cells cultivated
in vitro gives to these formerly lowly slaves of the
whole organism the immortality which they relinquished
when they performed their altruistic service in the body.
Carrel and many others that have come after him were
convinced that every somatic cell becomes freed from
death, if it is freed from the intact organism; the
long-term cultivation of a variety of "immortal" cell
lines supported this belief until the introduction of
modern karyology into these studies. Exact analysis
of the chromosomes of the well-known permanently
proliferating cell lines showed that these cells were
abnormal, heteroploid or mixoploid, and in many cases
had properties more or less characteristic of malignant
tissue. It became apparent that it would be necessary
to work with cells that were more nearly normal. This
criterion was met with the human diploid cell lines, as
described by Hayflick and Moorhead (1961).* These cells
have a fibroblast-like morphology and retain, in culture, a number of characteristics of normal cells, including a stable normal diploid karyotype.

With the introduction of these diploid cultures,
the question of cell mortality or immortality arose
again, this time not merely as an object of speculation, but as an object of experimental analysis. In
1961, these same authors reopened the discussion of
the immortality of cell cultures by showing that these
human fibroblasts have a limited lifespan. That is,

*L. Hayflick and P.S. Moorhead, Exp. Cell Res. 37: 614, 1961.

after a certain number of divisions, the population
must either degenerate and die, or become transformed
into a cell line which is potentially immortal, heteroploid, and in most cases displays characteristics of
malignant cell lines. Hayflick advanced the hypothesis
that even in vitro, normal cells do not escape death,
and that the possible reason for this obligatory decay lies
in the gradual accumulation of random damage to its nuclear
material.

With these views, Hayflick undoubtedly brought new
inspiration to the the then declining research into
aging using tissue and cell culture methods. After
the first flurry of papers, which dealt with the properties of various diploid cell lines, with the characteristics of their aging, and with the phenomena of
transformation and the nature of the transforming agents,
new puzzles began to emerge and new controversies began to crystallize. First of all, the correlation, or
lack thereof, between cell ploidy, malignancy, and
limited lifespan are not completely clear: diploid cells
are known which live longer than expected; there are
diploid cells which display malignant characteristics
and heteroploid cells which do not; and there are animal species whose cells readily become transformed
while the cells of other species appear to prefer death
to transformation. On the other hand, diploid cells in
culture which age as expected do show the same pattern
of morphologic and metabolic changes which occur when
they age in vivo.

Today, I have the honor and great pleasure to wel-
come scientists from different laboratories in Europe

and the United States who have come to summarize
their studies on the aging of cells in culture and to
stress those points which they consider worthy of
special attention. It is most unfortunate that
Professor Hayflick was not able to join us. Our discussion, of course, cannot cover the entire field of
aging in vitro; two areas of research have been omitted,
namely, aging in organ culture and the behavior of
cultured cells in relation to regeneration. The near
future will, we hope, bring much new information to
bear on these questions and more meaningful discussions
concerning them can then take place.

In today's program Dr. Hay intends to discuss some
of the various factors affecting the life span of diploid avian cells and some of the similarities and differences between their aging in vivo and in vitro.
Then Dr. Simons will describe the increased heterogeneity of cell size and its correlation with aging.
Dr. Soukupová will demonstrate a similar heterogeneity
in cell structure and activity in primary explant fragments. She will also try to show that even the simple
approach of measuring the latent period is still useful in determing different characteristics of aging.

Drs. Kritchevsky, Cristofalo, Macieira-Coelho and
Michl are all interested in the biochemical aspects
of aging in cell culture. Dr. Kritchevsky will discuss
lipid metabolism as a parameter of cellular aging; Dr.
Cristofalo will present data which reflect the relationships between aging in culture and energy metabolism,
nucleic acid content, and lysosomal enzyme activity.
Drs. Macieira-Coelho and Michl both have a particular

interest in nucleic acid metabolism. Dr. Macieira-Coelho
will discuss the relationship between cell growth kinetics
and the division cycle in cultures derived from adult
and embryonic tissues, while Dr. Michl will consider
the relationship between the growth-promoting α-globulin
fraction of serum and the synthesis of pyrimidines during
aging.

Professor Stanek's movie terminates the program
showing how unhappy a dying cell looks and how it is
surrounded and digested by its fellow cannibals of the
cultured population.

Emma Holečková

Žinkovy, Czechoslovakia
May 8, 1969

CELL STRAIN SENESCENCE IN VITRO: CELL CULTURE ANOMALY OR AN EXPRESSION OF A FUNDAMENTAL INABILITY OF NORMAL CELLS TO SURVIVE AND PROLIFERATE

ROBERT J. HAY

Carnegie Institution of Washington
Department of Embryology
115 West University Parkway
Baltimore, Maryland 21210

Since the advent of enzymic dissociation methods for the serial propagation of cells in culture numerous studies have detailed the changes in growth properties and morphology which take place with continued passage. Swim and associates [1, 2] clearly defined the characteristics of two distinct classes of cells which proliferate in vitro. One class, later termed primary cell lines by Harris [3] and others, comprises the apparently unaltered progeny of cells derived by dissociation of a given animal tissue. The second class, the so-called permanent cell lines, evolves during serial propagation of primary lines. We will be concerned mainly with the growth properties of primary cell lines in this discussion.

The observation that primary cell lines often have a limited survival time in vitro has been of considerable interest to cell biologists during the past 10 to 15 years. Two general hypotheses explaining this phenomenon have been proposed. The first suggests that current techniques of cell culture, especially the environment, are not adequate to permit continued proliferation and survival of primary cell types [1, 2, 4, 5, 6]. The second proposal implies that limited survival is intimately associated with the number of divisions undergone and is related in some way to senescence in the whole animal [7, 8, 9].

I propose to review some pertinent reports of work with cell lines from a variety of species, stressing the substantial role

which environment plays in the survival of primary cells in vitro.
The alternatives presented in the title of this article cannot be
resolved definitively from the evidence to be discussed. Nevertheless, it seems important to draw attention to the dramatic
changes in cell survival effected by alterations in culture
conditions since they may provide clues to explain the cause of
this degenerative phenomenon.

I will begin by outlining our own work with fibroblasts
isolated from skeletal muscle of embryonic chicks [5, 6]. The
growth span of six typical strains isolated from embryos of two
different ages is shown in Figure 1. A constant inoculation

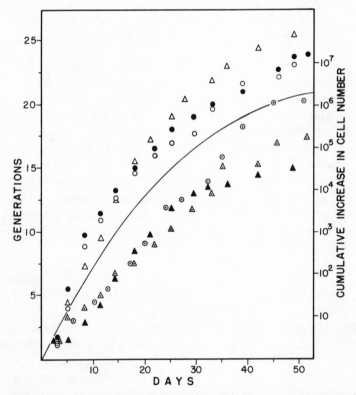

Fig. 1. Growth span of six typical cell strains isolated
from 10- to 12-day-old embryos (circles) or 18- to
20-day-old embryos (triangles). Generations = population
doublings.

density of 10^6 cells per 4 ounce prescription bottle was used at each subcultivation. Eagle's minimum essential medium supplemented with 10% calf serum and 5% embryo extract was used unless otherwise indicated.

Active cell proliferation occurred during the first 3 to 4 weeks but thereafter the rate of division declined progressively. Some strains achieved a maximum of about 25 doublings during the culture period of 50 to 60 days. We did not find any significant difference in the growth properties of strains from 10- to 12-day-old embryos versus 18- to 20-day-old embryos.

As shown in Figure 2, there was a marked decrease in the number of cells per unit of surface area at confluence during continued subcultivation. This suggests that chick cells become increasingly sensitive to contact inhibition, at least under the conditions here imposed. The presence of increased amounts of

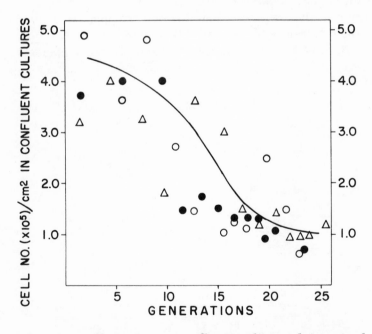

Fig. 2. Cell number in confluent cultures determined as a function of number of generations in vitro.

cell debris and a wide range of heterogeneity in cell shape was
also apparent in cultures at the later passage levels.

Using the same culture conditions, we now varied the
inoculation density and determined the growth span or survival
time (Fig. 3).   The growth rate diminished at the higher inoculation
levels due, presumably, to contact inhibition, especially during
the later stages of the culture regime.   Furthermore, the number
of doublings obtained decreased with increasing inoculation density.
After 32 days, the strain subcultivated at 3×10^6 cells per vessel
could no longer be maintained at that inoculation level.   That is,
we could not recover 3×10^6 cells to continue subcultivation.
The cells which were recovered, like those maintained at 10^6
and 2×10^6, had a very slow growth rate and were "senescent"
in morphology.   It is interesting to note that Hayflick [8] obtained
qualitatively similar results with human diploid fibroblasts.
Cultures subcultivated at a 2:1 split reportedly went through 40
population doublings while sister cultures subcultivated at a 10:1
split went through 57 doublings before phase III.   The total
calendar time involved was the same for both groups.   One can
argue that the difference 40 versus 57 is significant since sister
cultures, unlike cells from different strains or frozen ampules,

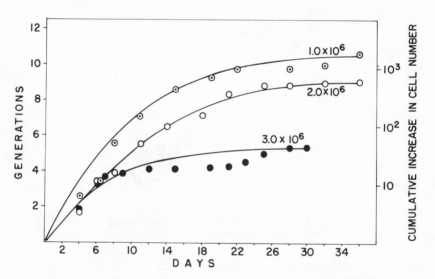

Fig. 3.   Influence of inoculation density on growth span.

are said to undergo very nearly the same number of population doublings [10].

The above findings suggested the possibility that the finite survival time is not related directly to the number of generations undergone. I should point out that although it has been suggested that the doubling potential of human cell strains is limited [7, 8], there is no published evidence which clearly differentiates between limited division potential and limited survival time. Attempts were made, therefore, to distinguish between these by a more direct experimental test. We isolated cells from embryonic chick muscle as usual and allowed the cultures to become confluent. We then added an overlay of the usual growth medium but now with 1.5% agar to keep the monolayer of stationary cultures intact during the repeated medium renewals to follow. The parent strain was subcultivated at 10^6 cells per vessel as before. Sister cultures were used at regular intervals, after removal of the agar overlay, to provide cells for substrains. The results, presented in Figure 4, showed that the growth span of these substrains (II to V) decreased with the time of maintenance in stationary culture.

One assumption involved in this type of experiment was that the cells maintained under the overlay were not actively proliferating. This was tested by labeling a number of cultures, companion to those used in the experiment of Figure 4, with tritiated thymidine. The label was added during the first six days in culture and was removed before addition of the agar overlay. The change in specific activity of DNA extracted at various intervals thereafter is shown in Figure 5.

It is apparent that there was some cell division, especially during the first week under the overlay. However, the extent of division, estimated by the change in specific activity of DNA extracted from labeled cultures, cannot account for the marked reduction observed in the growth span of substrains. Hence we concluded that the total time during which cells are maintained in monolayer culture is of utmost importance in limiting proliferation and survival.

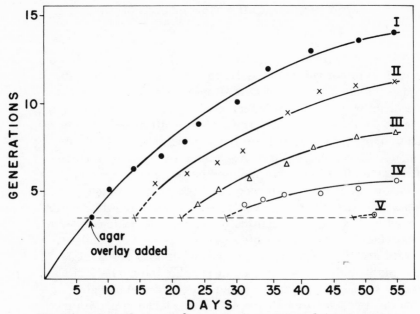

Fig. 4.   Growth span of parent strain (I) and 4 substrains
(II-V) initiated after various times in stationary culture.
Cultures under agar were fed 3 times per week.   Strains
were fed every 3-4 days and were subcultured when
confluency was reached.   Variability of cell populations
used to initiate substrains, estimated by erythrocin B,
decreased from 80-90% at day 7 to 40-60% at day 46.
Viability after cell strain establishment was 80-90%.

The above results are consistent with the hypothesis that
the culture environment is not adequate to permit long-term
survival of primary cells in vitro. One could postulate that
toxic substances, as yet undefined, accumulate in or on cells
in culture and that this eventually causes their degeneration.
Alternatively continual exposure of primary cells to a medium
containing suboptimal levels of essential nutrient or growth
factors could lead ultimately to the deterioration observed.   This
might result, for example, from environmentally induced error
in the synthesis of proteins involved in the transcription process.
This interesting concept was suggested by Orgel [11] as a
possible explanation for cellular deterioration associated with
aging but could apply in this situation even if natural cellular
aging is not involved.

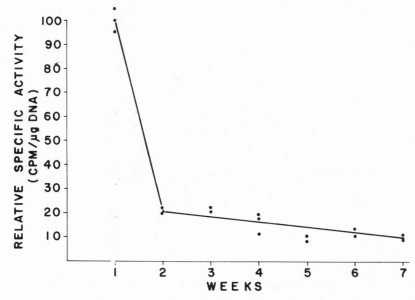

Fig. 5. Change in specific activity of DNA from cell
monolayers of cultures maintained for various times
in stationary culture.

One possible objection to these experiments employing an
agar overlay is that the agar itself might act on the cells to
decrease their growth potential. While the technique was chosen
because of its widespread use in virus assay methods [12] and in
organ culture [13], no other study of the long-term effects of agar
on cultured cells has been reported. Further studies with other
cell systems and maintenance techniques are required to clarify
this point.

More recently (Fig. 6) we have compared the growth span of
chick muscle fibroblasts in different media. One strain was
isolated and subcultivated under essentially the same conditions
as were used previously. An exception was that the embryo
extract was prepared in a more refined manner. We used
hyaluronidase to clarify the preparation and higher speed ultra-
centrifugation so the final product was clear [14]. The growth
span obtained was similar to that of the most vigorous strains
isolated previously [5].

In marked contrast, however, if cells from the same initial pool were grown in an improved medium, both the survival time and the number of generations attained were considerably increased. The improved medium consisted of Eagle's minimum essential medium but it was now supplemented with the same batch of calf serum at reduced concentration (5%) and with 5% tryptose phosphate broth instead of embryo extract. It is interesting that the strain which showed the highest initial proliferation rate, in medium with embryo extract, had the lowest total growth potential. While this experiment suggests again that inadequate environment plays a major role in the phenomenon of growth limitation, we must also consider the possibility that cell selection may be involved. Thus one could argue that the improved medium simply selected a different cell type with higher growth potential. This possibility can probably be tested by performing similar studies with cloned cell strains.

Note that in spite of the improved culture conditions, the proliferation rate of these chick cell strains did ultimately decline. However, it has been shown recently that this may not be a property of cells from all gallinaceous birds. Coon [15] reported isolating a fibroblast-like cell line from goose cartilage. This has undergone well over 150 doublings with no sign of growth decline. Whether this reflects a basic difference in response of cells from these two species to culture environment or selection of an altered cell type remains to be determined.

I would like now to discuss evidence, reported from several different laboratories, indicating that the growth span of human fibroblasts is also affected very dramatically by selection of different media. The early work of Swim and Parker [1] demonstrated this very clearly. A typical strain, isolated from human foreskin, showed very active proliferation for over 5 months and about 25 subcultures. The growth index then dropped somewhat and the strain reportedly went through about one population doubling per week until it eventually died out after 18 months in vitro. The total number of doublings undergone during this period cannot be determined accurately from the data provided but was certainly in excess of 100. Very striking differences in the growth span were observed when the composition of the medium was altered. The optimal growth span was obtained with medium F-15 which consisted of 5% filtered bovine embryo extract, 10% normal horse serum and 85% solution V-614.

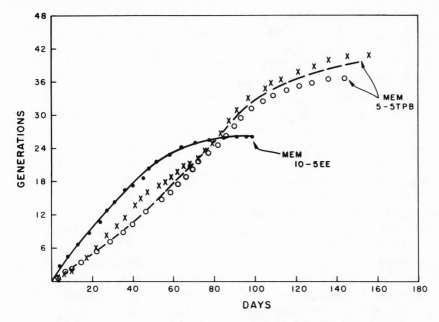

Fig. 6. Growth span of chick muscle fibroblasts in two
different media. Strains represented by dark circles
and by crosses were established from the same initial
cell pool. The strain indicated by open circles was
from a separate pool of cells.

MEM 10-5EE = Eagle's minimum essential medium
supplemented with 10% calf serum and 5% embryo
extract.

MEM 5-5TPB = Eagle's minimum essential medium
supplemented with 5% calf serum and 5% tryptose
phosphate broth (Difco).

Puck et al. [4] also favored the hypothesis that limited
survival of human fibroblasts was due to imperfections in
methodology or nutrition. Stringent precautions were therefore
adopted, including precise control of temperature and pH, gentle
trypsinization and the use of selected batches of serum. Strains
of euploid human fibroblasts were maintained for 10-12 months
using these techniques. In contrast, Puck et al. [4] refer to
experiments performed using earlier cultivation procedures
which yielded highly aneuploid human lung cells after only 2
months in vitro.

The extensive studies of Hayflick and Moorhead [7] and
Hayflick [8] effectively ruled out the possibility that chance
inclusion of toxic factors in the growth medium is responsible
for the onset of growth decline of human fibroblast strains.
Evidence excluding this possibility was derived from a variety of
experiments. Cell strains at early passage levels were able to
proliferate vigorously in the same pool of medium in which late
passage cells were entering the degenerate phase. Mixed
populations consisting of late passage male cells and earlier
passage female cells were found, after continued subcultivation,
to yield cells of the female type only. These and other similar
experiments lead to the suggestion that the composition of the
medium used plays no role in explaining the phenomenon of
limited cell division. It was suggested that the growth medium
and culture conditions used were entirely adequate [7, 8, 9].
At the same time, the novel hypothesis was advanced that this
phenomenon may be a manifestation at the cellular level of in vivo
senescence. Interesting results from part of the more recent
studies [8] are summarized in Table I. The average growth
span of 13 fibroblast strains from human fetal lung was 48
doublings whereas that of 8 strains from human adult lung was
only 20 population doublings. Note that the difference in doubling
potential was highly significant under the conditions imposed,
namely a 2:1 split ratio subcultivation regime using Eagle's
basal medium supplemented with 10% calf serum.

Although chance use of toxic batches of medium can be
excluded as the cause of degeneration of primary cell lines, the

Table I.   Growth Span of Human Fibroblast Strains
           from Fetal Versus Adult Lung

Donor Type	No. of Strains	Average No. of Subcultivations at 1:2 Split before onset of Phase III	Total Range
Fetal	13	48	35–63
Adult	8	20	14–29

Eagle's basal medium with 10% calf serum

Summarized from Hayflick [8].

possibility that inadequate overall culture conditions are involved
clearly has not been ruled out. As noted above, human fibroblasts
grown in a complex medium undergo in excess of 100 generations
[1] whereas strains maintained in Eagle's basal medium undergo
only 50 doublings [7, 8, 9]. Todaro et al. [16] were also able to
obtain a greater number of cell generations using Dulbecco's
modification of Eagle's basal medium and a constant inoculation
density at each subcultivation. Their results are summarized
in Table II. Note that in this small series the results were
similar for cells derived from either fetal or adult tissues.

Table II. Growth Span of Human Fibroblast Strains
from Fetal Lungs and Adult Skin (Biopsy)

Donor Type	No. of Substrains	Average No. of Cell Generations Obtained Before Growth Ceased	Total Range
Adult Skin	5	67	53-76[+]
Fetal Lung	4	64	53-73

Dulbecco's modification of Eagle's Basal Medium with
10 or 30% calf medium

Summarized from Todaro, Wolman and Green [16].

Table III. Effect of Serum Albumin Addition on the Growth Span
of Fibroblasts from Adult Skin

Medium Supplement	No. of Average Cell Generations Obtained Before Growth Ceased	Approx. Time in Culture (days)
10% Calf Serum	53	200
30% Calf Serum	65	200
10% Calf Serum + Serum Albumin (20 mg/ml)	100[+]	540[+]

Dulbecco's modification of Eagle's Basal Medium

Summarized from Todaro and Green [17].

Todaro and Green [17] reported findings, which are particularly revealing, of a direct study of the effects of addition of serum albumin to medium supporting the growth of human diploid fibroblasts. The results, summarized in Table III clearly indicate that active growth of euploid human fibroblasts can be extended for more than 100 generations during an interval of 18 months by employing this simple modification.

Let us now consider the growth characteristics of primary cell strains from the mouse and rat. Rothfels et al. [18] determined the growth properties of primary strains of embryonic mouse cells. The frequency of mitoses and changes in chromo-some pattern were observed with successive passage in vitro. The results, shown in Figure 7, indicate that the proliferation

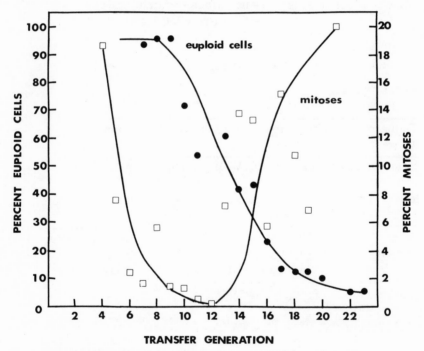

Fig. 7. Changes in percentage of mitoses and euploidy during transition of a primary to a permanent cell line. Data obtained from a strain of mouse embryonic cells (line 4) subcultivated about twice weekly. (From Rothfels et al. [18].

rate decreased with continued passage. After about 10 passages, by which time proliferation was minimal, the proportion of euploid cells also began to decrease. In similar experiments attempts were made to prolong the survival of euploid strains through the use of irradiated feeder cells. These were added with cells of the primary strain, at each subcultivation. Interestingly, the cell strain cultivated in this manner could be maintained at a higher proliferation rate for comparatively longer periods. Substrains deprived of the feeder system after various transfer generations rapidly become aneuploid (Fig. 8).

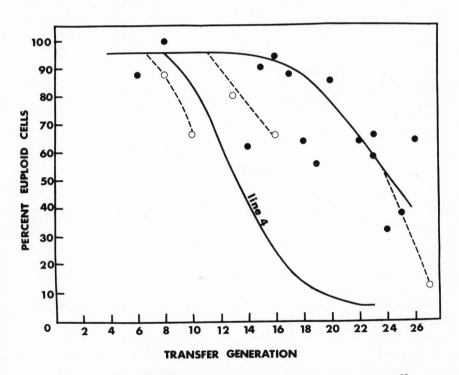

Fig. 8. Decrease in euploidy for mouse embryonic cell strain number 1 (solid line, closed circles) cultivated with feeder cells; substrains (broken line, open circles) taken off feeder at sixth, twelfth, and twenty-fourth transfer generation; and mouse embryonic cell strain (line 4) cultivated without feeder cells (compare with Fig. 7). (From Rothfels et al. [18]).

A considerable number of reports are now available indicating
that euploid rat cell strains may be maintained indefinitely in vitro
if adequate nutritional conditions are employed (Table IV).

Table IV.   Summary of Reports of Propagation of Diploid Rat
            Strains in Culture

Tissue of Origin	Time and No. of Passages	Additional Comments	Source
Rat embryos	22 months and 50+ passages	No sign of growth rate decline. Dependent on type of medium.	19
Adult Rat Skeletal Muscle Biopsy	15 months, 88 passages, 380+ generations	Early phase of growth decline but recovery	21
Myogenic strain from Neonatal Rat	More than 1 year, isolated by repeated cloning	No sign of growth decline, forms cross-straited muscle	22, 23
Liver of 2- to 5-week-old Rats	More than 1 year and over 100 doublings. Isolated by cloning	No sign of growth decline. Produces some characteristic serum proteins	24, 25

Petursson et al. [19] isolated a diploid cell strain from rat embryos
which underwent rapid proliferation for at least 22 months and
showed no sign of growth decline.   They indicated that chromosome 4
of these cells had upper biarms resembling satellites but such is
also observed in vivo in this species [20].   The culture medium
consisted of a mixture of N-15 and NC TC-109 with 15% bovine
serum all in saline G.   It is interesting and important to note that
cells from the same original pool which were grown only in
Eagle's basal medium supplemented with 15% bovine serum,
became heteroploid.

Krooth et al. [21] also isolated a euploid strain of rat cells with high proliferative activity. This was subcultivated over 88 times with 380 average cell generations. No sign of eventual growth decline and no change in karyotype could be detected. It should be emphasized that no selection method such as clonal isolation was used in either of the above studies.

More recently Yaffe [22, 23] has isolated a diploid cell line from rat skeletal muscle which survived for at least one year and retained the capacity to form normal myotubes in vitro. Coon [24] also reported isolating a diploid cell line which expressed some differentiated functions. In this case the source was rat liver and the cell line was able to synthesize some specific serum proteins as well as liver-specific enzymes. Coon has reportedly been able to maintain this line for more than one year, through well over 100 doublings and it still has shown no signs of growth decline [24, 25]. Clonal isolation methods were employed in these latter studies.

The crucial question with regard to the demonstration of apparently unlimited growth potential with these euploid rat cell strains has to do with the possibility that a malignant or pre-malignant change, not evident by karyotype analysis, has occurred during growth in vitro. Thus, Krooth et al. [21] observed a decrease in growth rate commencing 32 days after isolation of their euploid rat cell strain. About two weeks later a gradual upturn in proliferation rate ensued. It is conceivable that this change could reflect the occurrence of an alteration in cell properties similar to that which occurs with mouse cell strains but without concomitant development of aneuploidy. However, there is no substantial evidence to support this contention. Furthermore, this type of change in proliferation was not reported by the other investigators. Detailed studies of the growth characteristics and invasive potential of similar euploid strains at various times after isolation could be extremely enlightening at this point.

The above discussion of results from studies with cell strains from various species gives rise to several related questions. Each seems of major significance for resolution of the alternative

hypotheses suggested to explain the phenomenon of limited cell
proliferation in vitro.

Current culture conditions have been developed largely as a
result of the nutritional requirements of permanent cell lines.
Is it not plausible, therefore, that further refinements in the
nutritional and biophysical culture environment, adopted as a
result of studies with primary lines, may lead to prolonged
survival and proliferation of these cell types ?

Does the apparent ability of diploid rat cells to proliferate
indefinitely in vitro reflect a subtle pre-malignant change, or a
fundamental difference in the response of cells from this species
to culture conditions in current use ?

What are the underlying biochemical mechanisms responsible
for the difference in growth potential between primary and
permanent cell lines in species where this distinction applies ?

Is the phenomenon of limited proliferation and survival in
vitro related in any way to the apparently limited transplantability
of tissue cells in vivo [26, 27], and if so, is this in turn related
to aging of the whole animal ?

SUMMARY

In summary, evidence is available, especially from studies
with human and chick cells, suggesting that the survival of primary
strains is not necessarily associated with the number of divisions
undergone. Changes in the environment affect both survival time
and division potential very extensively but unlimited survival has
not yet been demonstrated with diploid cells from these species.
In marked contrast, however, certain diploid cell lines from rat
tissues seem to have the ability to survive indefinitely. This
appears to depend, at least in part, on the medium used. The
significance of these findings is discussed with reference to the
alternative explanations for cell strain senescence in vitro.

REFERENCES

1. H. E. Swim and R. F. Parker, "Culture characteristics of human fibroblasts propagated serially," Am. J. Hyg., 66: 235, 1957

2. H. E. Swim, "Microbiological aspects of tissue culture," Ann. Rev. Microbiol., 13: 141, 1959.

3. M. Harris, Cell Culture and Somatic Variation, New York, Holt, Rinehart and Winston, 1964.

4. T. T. Puck, S. J. Cierciura, and A. Robinson, "Genetics of somatic mammalian cells. III Long-term cultivation of euploid cells from human and animal subjects," J. Exp. Med., 108: 945, 1958.

5. R. J. Hay and B. L. Strehler, "The limited growth span of cell strains isolated from the chick embryo," Exp. Geront., 2: 123, 1967.

6. R. J. Hay, R. A. Menzies, H. P. Morgan, and B. L. Strehler, "The division potential of cells in continuous growth as compared to cells subcultivated after maintenance in stationary phase," Exp. Geront., 3:35, 1968.

7. L. Hayflick and P. S. Moorhead, "The serial cultivation of human diploid cell strains," Exp. Cell Res., 25:585, 1961.

8. L. Hayflick,"The limited in vitro lifetime of human diploid cell strains," Exp. Cell Res., 37: 614, 1965.

9. L. Hayflick, "Cell culture and the aging phenomenon," in: Topics in the Biology of Aging, New York, Interscience, 1966, p. 83.

10. V. J. Cristofalo, "Metabolic aspects of ageing in euploid human cells," This volume and personal communication.

11. L. E. Orgel, "The maintenance of the accuracy of protein synthesis and its relevance to ageing," Proc. Natl. Acad. Sci., 49: 517, 1963.

12. P. D. Cooper, "The plaque assay of animal viruses," in: Methods in Virology, Vol. 3, New York, Academic Press, 1967, p. 244.

13. O. A. Trowell, "The culture of mature organs in a synthetic medium," Exp. Cell Res., 16: 118, 1959.

14. H. G. Coon, "Clonal stability and phenotypic expression of chick cartilage cells in vitro," Proc. Natl. Acad. Sci., 55: 66, 1966.

15. H. G. Coon, "An established cell line of fibrobroblasts from goose cells," Carnegie Institution Year Book, 67: 421, 1969.

16. G. J. Todaro, S. R. Wolman, and H. Green, "Rapid transformation of human fibroblasts with low growth potential into established lines by SV40," J. Cell. Comp. Physiol., 62: 257, 1963.

17. G. J. Todaro and H. Green, "Serum albumin supplemented medium for long-term cultivation of mammalian fibroblast strains," Proc. Soc. Exptl. Biol. Med., 116: 688, 1964.

18. K. H. Rothfels, E. B. Kupelwieser, and R. C. Parker, "Effects of x-irradiated feeder layers on mitotic activity and development of aneuploidy in mouse-embryo cells in vitro," Canadian Cancer Conference, 5: 191, 1963.

19. G. Petursson, J. G. Coughlin, and C. Meylan, "Long-term cultivation of diploid rat cells," Exp. Cell Res., 33:60, 1964.

20. W. W. Nichols, "Relationships of viruses, chromosomes and carcinogenesis." Hereditas, 50: 53, 1963.

21. R. S. Krooth, M. W. Show, and B. K. Campbell, "A persistent strain of diploid fibroblasts," J. Natl. Canc. Inst., 32:1031, 1964.

22. D. Yaffe, "Retention of differentiation potentialities during prolonged cultivation of myogenic cells," Proc. Natl. Acad. Sci., 61: 477, 1968.

23. D. Yaffe and C. Revivi, to be published.

24. H. G. Coon, "Clonal culture of differentiated rat liver cells," J. Cell Biol., 39: 29a, 1968.

25. H. G. Coon, personal communication.

26. L. Siminovitch, J. E. Till, and E. A. McCulloch, "Decline in colony-forming ability of marrow cells subjected to serial transplantation into irradiated mice," J. Cell. Comp. Physiol., 64: 23, 1964.

27. P. L. Krohn, "Transplantation and aging," in: Topics in the Biology of Aging, New York, Interscience, 1966, p. 125.

A THEORETICAL AND EXPERIMENTAL APPROACH TO THE
RELATIONSHIP BETWEEN CELL VARIABILITY AND AGING
IN VITRO *

J.W.I.M. Simons

Department of Radiation Genetics
University of Leiden
The Netherlands

Anyone working with diploid cells is familiar with
the phenomenon of the limited lifespan of cells in vitro.
According to the senescence theory, this limited lifetime
should reflect aging in vivo [1]. In contrast to the senescence theory an environmental theory has also been proposed, stating that conditions in vitro are insufficient
for sustaining cell growth indefinitely.

Although this distinction between a senescence
theory and an environmental theory may be valid, it is important to remember that senescence in vivo might also be
a consequence of inadequate environmental conditions; thus
in vivo, aging in itself at the cellular level might also
be due to a failure in the adaptation of the cells.

At the moment what is needed most to test the aging
hypothesis is a demonstration of a correlation between
age-dependent changes in cells in vivo and cellular changes
occurring in cultures in vitro. Criteria to be used for
such correlations should be of a general nature so as to
include as many aging processes as possible.

Data of the type needed for such an approach are
still scanty. Some experimental conditions are known to
influence the limited lifespan in vitro. In the first
place there is the finding that the number of doublings

*This work was carried out in part under the Association
of the University of Leiden with Euratom. Contract No.
052-64-BIAN, and was in part supported by a grant from
the Netherlands Organization for the Advancement of Pure
Research, (Z.W.O.).

depends upon the split ratio [1,2]. More population
doublings were obtained at a higher split ratio. This
phenomenon suggests that processes of interaction or selection of cells occur under confluent conditions. A
second observation is that the lifespan of human skin
fibroblasts in vitro depends upon the type of serum used,
heterologous serum being more harmful than homologous or
autologous serum [3]. This finding is correlated with
changes in the size distribution of the cells and suggests
the induction of instability into the cells by the environment. One problem arising from these findings is to determine whether the aging in vitro is due to processes of cell
selection or to the induction of cellular instability simultaneously in all cells of the cell population.

    In this paper, aging has been studied using diploid
embryonic heart cells of the marsupial Potorous tridactylis.
These cells are characterized by six pairs of chromosomes.
Each chromosome can be distinguished individually. Only
one batch of pooled calf serum was used for all experiments to avoid the introduction of interfering side effects
due to different serum batches. As the criterion for possible aging effects, the frequency distribution of cell
volumes was used. These frequency distributions were determined with a Coulter counter connected to a plotter [4].
This plotter records the frequencies of the cells in
twenty-two volume classes. The data from the plotter were
fed into an IBM computer; after logarithmic transformation
of the values of the cell volumes, the following parameters
were estimated: mean, standard deviation, skewness and
kurtosis. The cells were measured in the phase of logarithmic growth, two days after seeding. Only one strain of
embryonic heart cells from a female Potorous was used.
For each experiment six substrains were formed; and these
strains were cultured individually and measured at each
passage until senescence made further subculturing im-
possible. Two sets of six cell strains have been cultured
and measured in this way. The cell strains were cultured
in a 2:1 split ratio.

    The first set of six cell strains was followed from
the 15th to the 29th passage. This culture period lasted
83 days. After the 30th subcultivation, growth stopped
completely for all six cell strains. Surprisingly, these
six cell strains all behaved much in the same way. As a
rule all six cell strains showed an increase or a decrease
in parameter value at the same passage and the same general
trend of increase or decrease in parameter value over the

whole culture period was found in all six cell strains. This is shown for the mean cell volume in Figure 1. Because the behavior of these substrains was so similar, the data for all six strains have been pooled for each passage. The changes in the values of the four parameters in subsequent passages are drawn in figure 2.

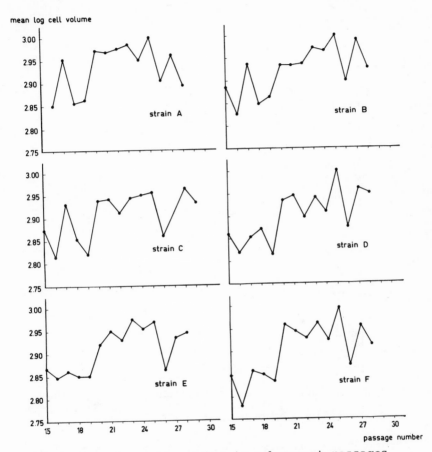

Fig. 1. Mean log cell volumes in subsequent passages of six cell strains (Potorous tridactylis embryonic heart cells).

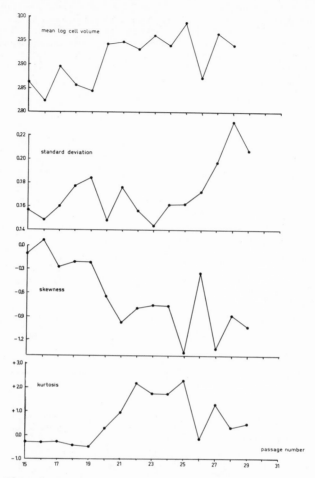

Fig. 2. Mean, standard deviation, skewness and kurtosis during the lifetime in vitro of Potorous tridactylis embryonic heart cells.

From the data in Figure 2 it can be noted that:

1. The overall trend in relation to increasing passage number is increase in mean volume, increase in standard deviation, decrease in skewness and increase in kurtosis.

2. A definite correlation exists between mean log cell volume, skewness and kurtosis. When the mean increases, the skewness decreases and the kurtosis increases. This shows that the changes in cell volume are not proportional to the cell volume. If the increase was in proportion to the cell volume, the skewness and kurtosis would remain the same. The increase in volume appears to be greater for the lower and medium volume classes giving rise to a negative skewness. As a result of the differential increase, relatively more cells are present in the medium volume classes, which is expressed as a positive kurtosis.

3. The standard deviation seems to be more or less independent of the other parameters.

4. Although overall changes exist in parameters with respect to subsequent passages, strong fluctuations in these parameters occur. It sould be kept in mind that these fluctuations are real and are not due to measuring errors, which are very small [4]. Figure 2 shows that a correlation has been found between cell aging and the parameters of the frequency distribution of cell volumes.

The second of six parallel cell strains was followed from the 12th to the 27th passage. This culture period lasted 56 days. In this experiment the cultures grew at a much faster rate than in the first experiment. The cultures were subcultured twice a week, while the cultures of the first experiment had several growth periods of seven days. After the 27th passage, growth stopped completely. Just as in the first series of cell strains, these six cell strains showed a surprising similarity in the pattern of their parameter values. Therefore the data for all six cell strains were again pooled. As a group the six cell strains of the second experiment did not behave exactly the same as the first group of six cell strains (Fig. 3).

Figure 3 suggests the following:

1. The overall trend in relation to successive passages is the same as in the first experiment: increase in mean volume, increase in standard deviation, decrease in skewness and increase in kurtosis.

2. In addition, in this experiment the mean and the skewness and the kurtosis are closely correlated in the same way as in experiment 1. Therefore, the type of alteration which occurs in the frequency distribution is much the same as in experiment 1.

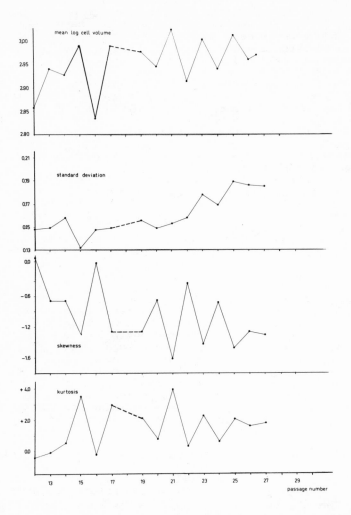

Fig. 3. Mean, standard deviation, skewness and kurtosis values during the lifetime of Potorous tridactylis embryonic heart cells. The data for passage 18 are missing.

3. As in the first experiment, large fluctuations in the cell volume parameters occur. The fluctuations here are even greater. In this experiment it is possible to correlate these fluctuations with culture conditions because there is a strict up-and-down pattern. Until the 26th passage these cell strains were subcultured twice a week and the growth periods were three and four days respectively. The length of these growth periods clearly have an influence on the size of the cells in the next passage two days after seeding. The subcultured cells show a larger volume two days after seeding when the preceding growth period was three days than when the preceding growth period lasted four days.

4. The relationship between the standard deviation and the other parameters is not obvious. In this experiment two conflicting tendencies seem to manifest themselves: from passage 23 onwards, the standard deviation is positively correlated with the mean volume, while from passage 13 to 17, there is a negative correlation.

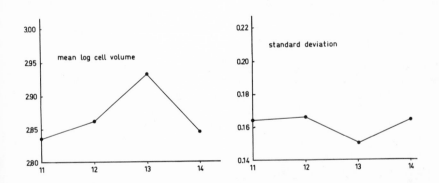

Fig. 4. Mean and standard deviation values during four early passages of Potorous tridactylis cells.

To see whether other cell populations at early passages show the same negative correlation between standard deviation and mean volume, in experiment 3 another six cell strains were cultured from the 11th to the 14th passage. As can be seen in Figure 4, there is also a negative correlation in this experiment.

In Figure 5 the relationship between mean volume and standard deviation of cell populations in early passages has been plotted. The data for all cell populations with a passage number lower than fifteen were used. The negative correlation between mean and standard deviation is obvious.

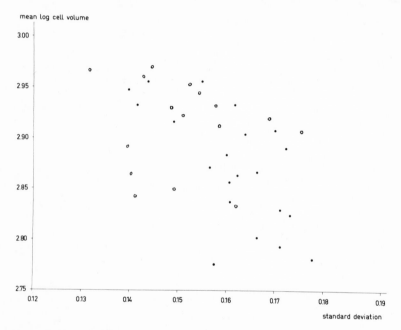

Fig. 5. Correlation between mean log cell volume and standard deviation of Potorous tridactylis embryonic heart cells during early passage.
    ● cell populations from experiment 2; passage 12-14
    o cell populations from experiment 3; passage 11-14

When the correlation between mean and standard deviation is negative for young cells and positive for old cells, the product of the standard deviation and the mean (m x̄ s) might be a better indicator for cell aging than each parameter alone. The fluctuations in young cells will be evened out, while the changes in old cells will become more obvious. This product (m x s) has been plotted in Figure 6 for all cell populations from experiments 1 and 2.

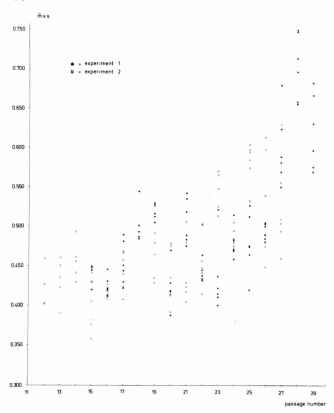

Fig. 6. Correlation of the product of mean and standard deviation (m x s) with passage numbers.
● data experiment 1.
o data experiment 2.

On the whole a gradual increase with passage number
can be seen. Aging phenomena seem to be present not only
during the last passage but even in passages where the cells
grow abundantly and look very healthy under the microscope.
Therefore, the increase (m x s) could be a useful indicator
of the physiological age of cell populations.

As a possible explanation for increase in mean cell
size with aging, an increase in the number of tetraploid
or other polyploid cells has been postulated [3]. In
Figure 7 chromosome counts are given for the six cell
strains of experiment 2. These counts were taken at passage 24, three passages before the end of the lifespan.
The cells of all six cell strains are still predominantly
diploid. The diploid number is 12. The percentage of
tetraploid cells is about 20, which is a normal value for
this cell strain [5]. The only difference from young cells
is the presence of a few triploid cells, which are very
rare in young cells. So it can be concluded that in these
Potorous strains, increase in the number of polyploid cells
did not occur during aging.

The data obtained from these experiments give rise
to some theoretical considerations about cell aging in
vitro. First, during cell aging there is an overall increase in mean volume and standard deviation. The fluctuations in these parameters rather indicate the induction
of changes in all cells simultaneously than processes of
the cell selection. Secondly, under these experimental
conditions cell aging is more directly correlated with
the number of population doublings than with time in culture. In experiment 1, 29 passages were obtained and in
experiment 2, 27 passages, while the time in culture from
the 15th passage amounted to 83 days for experiment 1 and
to only 46 days for experiment 2. Thirdly, since the life-
spans of the six parallel cell strains in each experiment
were identical, 29 passages for the cell strains in experiment 1, and 27 passages for the cell strains in experiment
2, it seems possible that the difference of two passages
in lifespan between the cell strains in the first and in
the second experiment is due to the faster growth rate in
experiment 2. This is confirmed by observations of cells
from experiment 2. By culturing cells from the 25th passage in growth periods of 10 days, four additional doublings could be obtained for all six cell strains. This
shows that a fast growth rate reduces the number of doublings and that the lifespan is not fixed, but may be extended under favorable conditions. Probably changing the

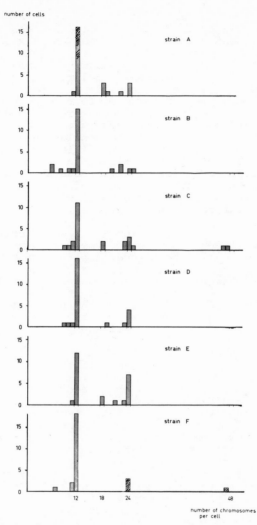

Fig. 7. Histograms of chromosome numbers in six cell strains of Potorous tridactylis embryonic heart at the 24th passage, three passages before the end of the lifespan. The diploid number is twelve.

lengths of growth periods also influences the parameter
values; this can be seen in Figure 8 where the mean values
of the product of mean and standard deviation (m x s) have
been given for experiments 1 and 2. In experiment 2,
where the growth periods were three and four days until
the 26th passage, (m x s) increases regularly; however,
in the first experiment, two big oscillations occur. There
the time between passages was three or four days until passage 21, after which the growth periods were seven days.
Thus an increase in the growth periods is correlated with
a decrease in (m x s), which could be considered a tempor-
ary beneficial effect on the cells, resulting in an extended lifespan. Therefore, this figure indicates that
the parameters obtained by size analysis can serve as useful indicators of the physiological age of the cell populations when the cells are cultured under strict constant
conditions throughout their whole lifespan.

A fourth important observation in these experiments is the simultaneous changing of the parameters of
the six independent cell strains over a period of nearly
three months. This implies that very strict rules exist,
which cause these changes. When even better standards for
culture conditions, for instance, by a constant growth period, have been achieved, the curves of the parameters will
probably show smaller fluctuations and will be even better
suited as indicators of physiological age.

It would be interesting to know whether it is possible to cancel out all fluctuations. In theory it is
quite possible that these fluctuations are partly due to
intrinsic factors in the cell and that under strictly
controlled conditions fluctuations in the size of the cells
would still occur due to these intrinsic factors. The
frequency distribution of cell volumes might reflect in
this way a control system for the regulation of processes
in the cell. The negative correlation between mean and
standard deviation indicates, that an increase in standard
deviation, which might reflect cellular disorganization,
might be counteracted by an increase in cell volume. In
this way a cell population in a constant environment may
show a continuous oscillation due to intrinsic factors.
During the lifespan such spontaneous oscillations might
be influenced by spontaneous intrinsic changes or by ex-
trinsic conditions to such an extent that the control
mechanism responsible for these oscillations is damaged
or destroyed; this is observed as cell aging.

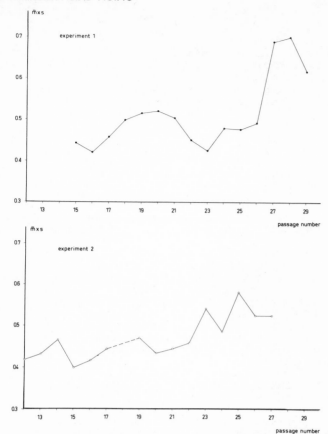

Fig. 8. Correlation of the product of mean and standard deviation (m x s) of experiment 1 and 2 with passage numbers.

        Although the distinction between intrinsic and ex-
trinsic factors is very important in relation to aging,
I believe that at present this distinction is not very
useful to the experimental approach. It is not known for
sure that cellular aging in vivo is due at least in part to
purely intrinsic factors only; extracellular factors may

play a role as well. More important at the moment are
the correlations between aging in vivo and aging in vitro.
This method of cell size analysis would provide an opportunity for investigating whether there exists in vivo
a similar correlation between cell size and age. This
could be established by measuring cell populations taken
from individuals of different age.

SUMMARY

        By means of size analysis of embryonic heart cells
of Potorous tridactylis, the following conclusions were
reached:

        1. Cell senescence of these cells is correlated with
increase in mean log volume, increase in standard deviation,
decrease in skewness and increase in kurtosis.
        2. Cell senescence in these strains is not correlated
with increase in polyploidy.
        3. Aging of these cells is correlated with number
of doublings rather than with time in culture.
        4. The number of doublings of these cells can be in-
creased by lengthening the growth periods between subcultivations.
        5. Parallel cultures of these cells agree very
closely in aging phenomena.

Furthermore, it appears that the method of cell size
analysis can produce useful criteria for the physiological
age of aging cells in vitro when the culture conditions
can be kept constant throughout the whole lifespan. The
data indicate induction of changes into all the cells
simultaneously rather than cell selection.

        As a possible interpretation it has been postulated
that a regulatory mechanism exists in the cell, which
counteracts disorganization in the cell by increase in
cell volume and that cell aging is due to disintegration
of this regulatory mechanism.

REFERENCES

1. L. Hayflick, "The limited in vitro lifetime of human diploid cell strains," Exp. Cell Res., 37:636, 1965.
2. S.J. Todaro, S.R. Wolman, H. Green, "Rapid transformation of human fibroblasts with low growth potential into established cell lines by SV_{40}," J. Cell. Comp. Phsy., 62:265, 1963.
3. J.W.I.M. Simons, "The use of frequency distributions of cell diameters to characterize cell populations in tissue culture," Exp. Cell Res., 45:336, 1967.
4. J.W.I.M. Simons, "Characterization of somatic cells by determination of their volumes with a Coulter counter." To be published.
5. H. Van Steenis, R.V. Tuscany, Personal communication.

CHANGES OF THE LATENT PERIOD OF EXPLANTED TISSUES DURING ONTOGENESIS

Milena Soukupová, Emma Holečková and
Přemysl Hněvkovský

Department of General Biology, Medical Faculty,
Charles University, Prague, Czechoslovakia

During the first fifty years of work with animal
tissues and cells cultured in vitro, it has been clearly
shown that the age of the donor determines the behavior
of the explants. There are two basic phenomena which
have been subjected to detailed experimental analysis.
The first of these to be studied was the latent period,
defined as the time after which cells first emigrate
out of a freshly explanted tissue fragment. This period
of dormancy increases with the increasing age of a normal tissue donor. The other phenomenon, which has been
known for about 10 years, is the limited lifetime of
diploid cells in culture. This lifespan is longer for
cells cultured from embryos than for cells cultured
from mature donors. Both phenomena have been studied
in our laboratory. This paper deals with our findings
concerning the relationship between the latent period
of fragment cultures from different rat organs and age.

As early as 1910, Carrel and Burrows [1,2,3] described the prolongation of the time required to overcome the stress of explantation when cultures were set

up from tissues of donors of increasing age. This
basic finding revealed two main problems: one is the
question of the mechanism responsible for this increase
of the latent period with donor age; the other is the
response of different cell types to aging.

Some twenty years ago, Doljanski and his co-workers
[4] tried to measure the latent period of a series of
explanted organs of young and adult chickens and came
to the conclusion that cells of all organs have latent
periods of uniform duration at a given ontogenetic stage.
In addition, they found that the latent period in
primary explants increased only during active growth of
the organism; after cessation of active growth, the
latent period did not go on increasing [5].

In our experiments with rats, we were unable to
confirm these results, which had been obtained in
chickens. Our studies included hanging drop cultures
of the brain, heart, liver, kidney and spleen of newborn
(1- to 3 -day-old), adult (8-to 12-month-old) and old
(21- to 24-month-old) rats. Ten explants were set up
from every organ and the latent period was estimated
indirectly, by counting the number of fragments with
migrating cells daily during 7 or more days of incubation at 36-37°C [6,7].

Figure 1 shows that, although the latent period increases for every organ studied, the organs behave in
different ways. Migrating cells appear sooner in explanted fragments of newborn rats, but even here, the
heart and brain show signs of lower activity (there are
less fragments with cell migrations and their latent

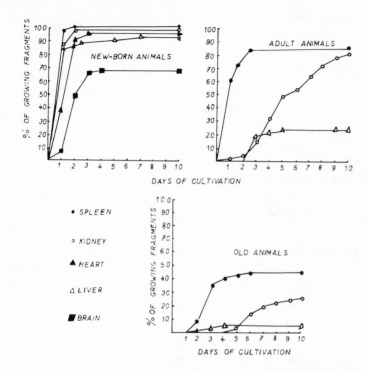

Fig. 1.   The latent period of the spleen,
kidney, heart, liver, and brain and the percentage of growing fragments (ordinate).
Days of cultivation (abscissa).

period is longer) than do the spleen, kidney and
liver explants. In adult rats, there is no cell migration in heart and brain under these culture conditions;
however, the three more actively growing organs have
begun to differentiate, the spleen being the most active
organ with the shortest latent period, followed by
kidney and then liver. In old rats, the duration of
the latent period increases further with no change in

the order of these three organs.

The findings on the tenth day were subjected to statistical analysis. There were significant differences not only between the groups of newborn and adult rats, but also between the groups of adult and old rats.

Our findings show first that the latent period increases in the rat after cessation of the active growth of the organism, and, second, that the increase in the latent period is not uniform for all the organs studied, but that differences exist in the duration of the latent period which are characteristic for each organ. A counterpart of these latter findings may be found in the results of Glinos and Bartlett [8] who measured the latent period of rat liver explants from newborn, adult, and old rats, and also found an increase from adult to old age. Different reactions of different organs of newborn rats to explantation were described recently by Zaroff and his co-workers [9]. These authors found significant differences in the plating efficiency of cells from the liver, kidney, spleen, bone marrow and thymus, and called the colony-forming cells "presumptive tissue culture cells." In these experiments, the differences appeared even among the cells from different organs of one donor. It seems that these findings represent additional evidence that the latent period increases during the entire period of ontogenesis, at least for organs containing cells capable of division, and that the time course of this increase

is different for different organs. The reasons for
this increase remain obscure.

Many authors who are interested primarily in the
macromolecular aspects of aging, look to the intercellular substances for clues to the mechanisms of cell
degeneration and cell loss from the tissues of aging
subjects. The quantitative, as well as the qualitative,
structure of the intercellular substances changes during
ontogenesis, and their increase in quantity together
with decreased permeability has been considered a cause
of cell damage in old age. Simms, Stillman, and their
group [10,11] presented evidence that in tissue cultures the latent period of adult tissues may actually
be shortened by enzymatic, trypsin digestion of the
tissue before explantation.

In order to investigate more closely the role of
the intercellular substances, we conducted a series of
experiments with trypsin-digested kidneys from young
and old rats. Kidney tissue of both young and old rats
was trypsinized simultaneously, the cells were collected,
and the yield of cells per unit of wet tissue weight
was calculated.

Figure 2 shows that the cell yield was always
greater in the young than in the old rats. The reason
for this difference may be either a greater cellularity
of the young kidney, or a lower sensitivity of the intercellular substances of the old animal's tissue to trypsin,
or both. When examined microscopically, the cells of
the old rats were always larger than those of the young
animals. Culture vessels from both suspensions, were
inoculated with the same number of cells [500,000 per

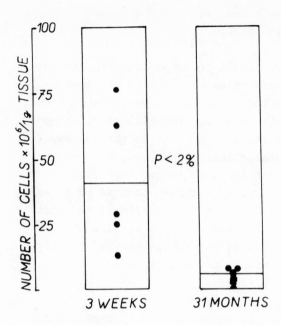

Fig. 2. The cell yield from 1 g of
kidney tissue of young (3 weeks) and
old (31 months) rats.

ml of medium] and then incubated for three weeks.

Figure 3 shows the results after two weeks of
cultivation, when cells of the young rats had already
formed a monolayer, but the cells of the old rats had
formed only a few degenerating colonies. One objection
to this experiment is the realization that the trypsin-
digested cells may still bear an envelope of extracellular collagen on their surface, and that the properties of this supposed envelope could be different in
young and old cells. Therefore, we subjected the

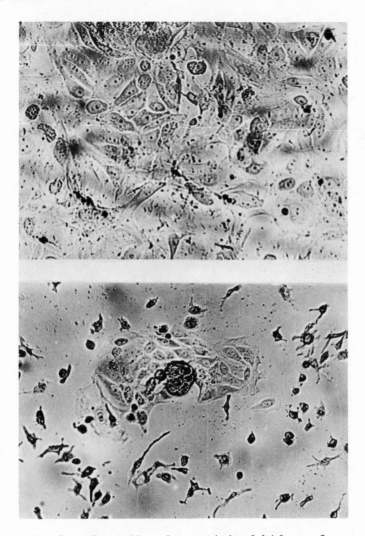

Fig. 3. The cells of trypsinized kidney of a
young (upper part) and an old (lower part) rat
after two weeks of cultivation.

trypsinized cells to the action of collagenase in order
to free the suspended cells from any collagen remnants,
and we cultured them again after this procedure.

Figure 4 shows the results of hydroxyproline analysis
on part of the material which we used for cultivation.   To
our surprise, a considerable amount of hydroxyproline was
present in both the trypsinized cell samples, but after the

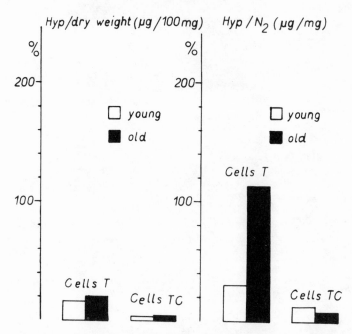

Fig. 4.   The amount of hydroxyproline expressed
as percentage (the amount of hydroxyproline in
the young rat's kidney tissue remaining after
trypsinization = 100%).   Cells T = cells collected
after trypsin treatment.   Cells TC = cells collected after trypsin and collagenase treatment.

action of trypsin and collagenase, the amount of hydroxyproline became negligible [12].

Figure 5 shows that the difference between the cells
obtained in this way from the kidneys of young and old
rats remained unchanged. The trypsin-collagenase treatment damaged the cells more than trypsinization alone,
but, again, the cells of the young rats were better able
to overcome this stress. They formed many colonies,
while in the same time period the cells of the old animals appeared as a few ghost-like elements.

Thus, the possible presence of extracellular substances on the surface of cultured cells does not directly
influence their behavior. Other facts also support
this conclusion; for example, there were small amounts
of extracellular substances present in the brain, which
nevertheless had the longest latent period of all the
organs studied [6,7].

The fragment cultures of kidney from old rats showed
very late cellular migration, i.e., one week or more
after explantation. Not only was the latent period
longer, but the migrating cells had a different appearance [13]. Figure 6 shows rich epithelial sheets
of the newborn rat kidney, containing small healthy-
looking cells with nuclei of uniform size. The cells
which appear in cultures from adult rat kidney have a
looser sheet of larger vacuolated cells with anisocyto-
sis and signs of pycnosis in some nuclei. Small, very
thin membranes growing out of the old rat kidney fragments bear signs of cellular damage, and a large amount

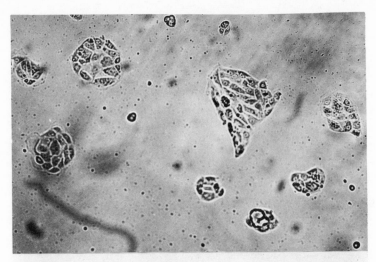

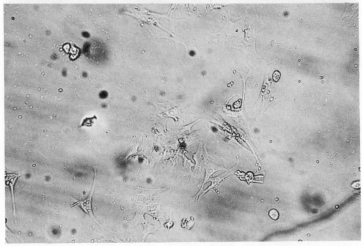

Fig. 5. The cells obtained from kidney
tissue of a young (upper part) and an old
(lower part) rat after trypsin and collagenase treatment. Photographed after 5 days
of cultivation.

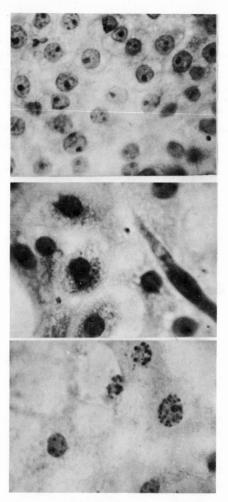

Fig. 6. Epithelial cells emi-
grating from kidney fragments
of newborn (upper part), adult
(middle part) and old (lower
part) rats.

of cytoplasmic vacuolation and karyorhexis. They live
and metabolize in the medium for a considerable time
before the first cells appear, and we wondered if this
changed medium could negatively influence the vitality
of the cells from older donors.   Therefore, we
studied [14] the influence of this changed medium by
comparing cultures of newborn and adult rat kidney.
First we prepared the explants from the adult rat kidney and waited until migrating cells appeared. This
usually happened on the 5th or 6th day of incubation.
We then opened the culture chamber and added a fresh
fragment of newborn rat kidney in the area of the
growing old animal tissue. After 24 hr of further incubation, we fixed and stained the adjacent cultures
with Harris' hematoxyline and examined their appearance.
The latent period of the newborn rat tissue was not influenced by the medium used by the old rat kidney and
rich epithelial sheets were present in all cases.
Similarly, the appearance of the cells was not changed;
the young cells retained their young appearance and
the old cells retained theirs.   Figure 7 shows such an
adjacent pair of explants, the young and the old one
being immediately recognizable. At a greater magnifi-
cation, a clear borderline was seen even in cases where
the two cell sheets met and joined together. In these
experiments, there were no signs of rejuvenation of the
old cultures or of cell hybridization.

The last point which seems to be of interest to us
is the great heterogeneity of the explants in later
stages of ontogenesis. In adult animals there are kidney fragments from which cells begin to migrate as early as
in newborn rats, other fragments, where it takes 2,3 or

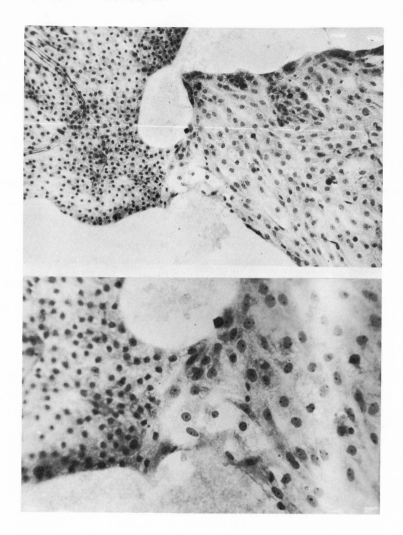

Fig. 7. Adjacent cultures of a newborn (left) and
an adult (right) rat kidney with confluent membranes.
In low (upper part) and high (lower part) magnifi-
cation.

more days before migration begins, and still others,
which remain completely inactive during the whole incubation period. Since technical reasons can be excluded, some biological explanation of this phenomenon
should be sought. The heterogeneity increases with increasing age, again at a different rate in different
organs. Our present hypothesis is that the number of
presumptive tissue culture cells or progenitor cells
decreases with age, and that the situation may still be
aggravated by extracellular factors causing cell damage
in situ, such as vascular insufficiencies or different
pathological processes. In any case while all the organs of the newborn rats contained a large quantity of
cells capable of migration and division, the organs of
older donors looked like a mosaic of tissue regions with
many, few or perhaps no cells capable of life in vitro.

REFERENCES

1. A. Carrel and M.T. Burrows, "Cultivation of adult tissues and organs outside of the body," J. Am. Med. Ass.,
   55:1379, 1910.
2. A. Carrel and M.T. Burrows, "Cultivation of sarcoma
   outside of the body," J. Am. Med. Ass., 55:1554, 1910.
3. A. Carrel and M.T. Burrows, "On the physicochemical
   regulation of the growth of tissues. The effects of
   the dilution of the medium on the growth of the spleen,"
   J. Exp. Med., 13:562, 1911.
4. L. Doljanski, J. Goldschmidt, and R. Hoffman, "Etude
   comparative sur la durée de la période de latence
   pour la croissance de différents tissus et organes
   d'une poule adulte in vitro," Compt. Rend. Soc. Biol.,
   126:744, 1937.

5. L. Doljanski, M. Palevitsch and J. Goldschmidt, "Etude comparative sur la durée de la période de latence pour la croissance de tissus adultes in vitro pendant différentes périodes du développement postembryonnaire," Compt. Rend. Soc. Biol., 133:56, 1940.

6. J. Michl, M. Soukupová, and E. Holečková, "Ageing of cells in cell and tissue culture," Exp. Gerontol., 3:129, 1968.

7. M. Soukupová and E. Holečková, "The latent period of explanted organs of newborn, adult and senile rats," Exp. Cell Res., 33:361, 1964.

8. A.D. Glinos and E.G. Bartlett, "The effect of regeneration on the growth potentialities in vitro of rat liver at different ages," Cancer Res., 11:164, 1951.

9. L. Zaroff, G. Sato, and S.E. Mills, "Single-cell platings from freshly isolated mammalian tissue," Exp. Cell Res., 23:565, 1961.

10. H.S. Simms and N.P. Stillman, "Substances affecting adult tissue in vitro. I. The stimulating action of trypsin on fresh adult tissue," J. Gen. Physiol., 20:603, 1937.

11. H.S. Simms and N.P. Stillman, "Substances affecting adult tissue in vitro. II. A growth inhibitor in adult tissue," J. Gen. Physiol., 20:621. 1937.

12. M. Soukupová, P. Hněvkovský, M. Chvapil, and Z. Hrůza, "Effect of collagenase on the behavior of cells from young and old donors in culture," Exp. Gerontol., 3:135, 1968.

13. M. Soukupová, "Cellular morphology of explanted spleen and kidney of newborn, adult and senile rats," Physiol. Bohemoslov., 14:107, 1965.

14. M. Soukupová, E. Holečková, and O. Cinnerová, "Behavior of explanted kidney cells from young, adult and old rats," Gerontologia 11:141, 1965.

LIPID METABOLISM IN HUMAN DIPLOID CELLS*

David Kritchevsky† and Barbara V. Howard‡

The Wistar Institute of Anatomy and Biology
Philadelphia, Pennsylvania

The human diploid cell lines presently available provide a unique system for studying human tissue at the cellular level. In addition, the limited capacity for doubling displayed by these cells has been interpreted as senescence at a cellular level. Hence, human diploid cells present an interesting system for the study of aging in vitro.

There is a relatively small number of published works on the synthesis and utilization of lipids by cultured cells. The fact that lipids are not required as nutrients in cell lines which can be grown in chemically defined medium [1] suggests that these cells can synthesize lipids. Direct synthesis of lipids by L cells grown in synthetic medium has been demonstrated by Bailey [2]. Lipid synthesis and utilization by cells grown in medium that contains

*Supported, in part, by USPHS Training Grant TI-GM-142 from the National Institute of General Medical Sciences, USPHS Career Award #4-K06-HE 00734 from the National Heart Inst. and Grant #R01-CA 10028 from the National Cancer Inst.
†Wistar Professor of Biochemistry, Division of Animal Biology, School of Veterinary Medicine, University of Pennsylvania, Philadelphia, Pennsylvania.
‡Present address: Dept. of Microbiology, University of North Carolina, Raleigh, North Carolina.

serum is more complicated. The lipids present in serum can
inhibit lipid synthesis [2] and synthesis may be spared by
the uptake of triglycerides [3], fatty acids [4], and cholesterol and cholesterol esters [5,6].

Our initial studies on the lipid spectra of young and
old WI-38 cells [7] indicated a surprisingly high level of
free (unesterified) fatty acids (FFA). There are few data
available concerning the FFA content of other cells and tissues. Therefore, we have examined the FFA content of various
cells and tissues, and have then proceeded to investigate the
possible sources of FFA in human diploid cells.

Finally, we have compared the lipids of the normal WI-38
cells with those of the line WI-38VA13A, which was derived
from WI-38 by transformation with SV40 virus [8]. This comparison provided us the opportunity to examine several possible changes in cell lipids following transformation.

MATERIALS AND METHODS

Starter cultures of strain WI-38 cells were obtained
from Dr. L. Hayflick, and cultures of WI-38VA13A cells were
obtained from Dr. A. Girardi of this institute. Both types of
cells were cultured as a monolayer in 2-liter Povitzky bottles containing 150 ml of medium. The growth medium consisted of Eagle's basal medium in Earle's balanced salt solution, supplemented with 10% calf serum and 50 μg/ml aureomycin. The gas phase, which was 10% CO_2 in air, maintained the
the pH between 7.0 and 7.4. The cultures were checked peri-
odically to insure the absence of mycoplasma contamination.

Routinely, the cells were subcultivated at 1:10 ratios,
and confluency was attained at about eight days under these
conditions. Cells were harvested from the glass surface
using an 0.25% buffered trypsin solution. The cells were
washed three times by centrifugation (500 x g for 3 min at
5°C) and resuspended in a phosphate-buffered balanced salt
solution (PBS), described by Cristofalo and Kritchevsky[9].
The washed cells were lyophilized and weighed. When not
used immediately, cells were stored at -5°C.

To extract lipid from the cells, weighed amounts of lyophilized cells were transferred to extraction thimbles (Whatman Fat Free) and extracted continuously with methanol: methylal (1:4) for 5 hr at 60°C in a Soxhlet extraction apparatus. The extract was washed with 1/5 volume of 0.05N NaCl and dried under nitrogen. The dry weight was taken as the total lipid of the cells.

Separation into neutral lipids and phospholipids was accomplished on a 10 g silicic acid column. The total lipid extract was dissolved in hexane and placed on the column. Neutral lipids were eluted with 200 ml chloroform and phospholipids with 200 ml methanol. The eluates were dried under vacuum and weighed. All samples were stored under nitrogen at -5°C.

Neutral lipids and phospholipids were subfractionated using thin layer chromatography (TLC) on activated Silica Gel G (Brinkmann). For optimum separation of neutral lipids aliquots of a chloroform solution were streaked on two separate (thin-layer) plates (250 μ thick). One plate was developed in petroleum ether:ethyl ether:acetic acid (85:15:1) to isolate cholesteryl esters, triglycerides and free fatty acids; the more polar neutral lipids remained at the origin. The second plate was developed in petroleum ether: ethyl ether:acetic acid (55:45:1) to separate fatty acids, cholesterol and di- and monoglycerides; the less polar lipids traveled with the solvent front. Appropriate standards were applied to each plate and positions of each fraction were fixed by exposure to iodine vapor. (Lipid classes were also identified by standard colorimetric procedures). The areas containing the various lipids were marked and, after sublimation of the iodine, the silicic acid area representing each lipid was carefully scraped off the plate and the lipids quantitated by the acid dichromate method of Amenta [10].

A methanolic solution of the phospholipid fraction was applied as a streak on a 500 μ-thick plate and subjected to development in chloroform:methanol:acetic acid:water (55:45:2:4). The component phospholipid fractions were marked by exposure to iodine vapor and identified by

comparison with appropriate standards. Phospholipid fractions were eluted from the silicic acid by sequential extraction with developing solvent (4 ml), developing solvent
(2 ml), methanol (2 ml), and methanol:acetic acid:water
(75:1:5) (2 ml). The combined eluates were evaporated to
dryness and phosphorus was determined by the method of
Fiske and Subbarow [11].

Fatty acid methyl esters were prepared from total neutral lipid or phospholipid fractions by saponification and
diazomethylation. Saponification was carried out at 70°C
for 4 hr in 3 ml 60% ethanol and 2 ml 10N NaOH. Nonsaponi-
fiables were removed by extraction with petroleum ether.
After acidification of the aqueous phase, fatty acids were
extracted using ethyl ether. Diazomethane was generated by
the method of James [12] and distilled directly into the
fatty acid-ether solution. The ether was then evaporated
and the methyl esters stored under N_2 at -5°C.

Gas liquid chromatography was performed on a column
containing 15% ethylene glycol succinate on 100-120 mesh
gas chrom P (Glowall Corp., Willow Grove, Pa.). An Argon
ionization detector was used. The column was standardized
for retention times and quantitated at 160°C and 20 psi
using purified methyl esters (Hormel Institute, Austin,
Minn.). The fatty acids were quantitated by measuring the
areas under each peak and comparing them to standard curves
that had been constructed for each fatty acid.

Of the cells used for FFA analysis, the WI-38VA13A
cells, muscle fibroblasts, HeLa, L and L-5178Y cells were
obtained from Drs. L. Hayflick, A. Girardi, M. Fogel,
R. Carp, C. Gauntt, and G. Rothblat, respectively, all of
the Wistar Institute. A strain of skin fibroblasts was
obtained from Dr. W. Mellman of the Hospital of the University of Pennsylvania. The WI-38, WI-38VA13A, skin and
muscle fibroblasts and HeLa cells were cultured as monolayers on Eagle's basal medium using methods described previously. The L cells were cultivated both as a monolayer
and in suspension, and they could be routinely alternated
from one method of culture to the other; L-5178Y cells were

cultivated only in a suspension culture. For the suspension cultures, cells were agitated in Joklik's modification of Eagle's basal medium (Grand Island Biological Co., Grand Island, New York) supplemented with 10% calf serum and 50 μg/ml aureomycin. In certain of the studies fetal calf serum (Microbiological Associates, Bethesda, Maryland) was used in place of calf serum (Flow Laboratories, Rockville, Maryland) and the concentrations were varied from 2 to 10%. Cells were harvested and washed using procedures described previously, except that the trypsin was omitted in harvesting the suspension cultures [7].

Rat tissues were obtained from 200 g male Wistar rats which had been fed a normal diet.

Isolation and Quantitation of Free Fatty Acids

The procedure developed for the isolation and quantitation of free fatty acids is summarized below. An aliquot of the harvested cells was taken for the determination of dry weight of cell protein. The remainder was extracted with 20 volumes of warm chloroform:methanol (2:1) for 15 min. This total lipid extract was washed with 1/5 volume of 0.05N NaCl according to the procedure of Folch et al. [13]. Phospholipids were removed from the lipid extract by the method of Bloor [14]. The total lipid extract was dried under a stream of N_2 and redissolved in 2 ml of cold petroleum ether in a centrifuge tube. Seven ml of cold acetone and 3 drops of a saturated solution of $MgCl_2$ in ethanol were added, and the tubes placed in an ice bath for 5 min. The samples were then centrifuged for 10 min at high speed in an International centrifuge and the precipitate was washed once with 2 ml acetone. The efficiency of the precipitation was assayed by adding a mixture of ^{14}C-labeled phospholipids to the cell lipid extract, and the results indicated that more than 96% of the phospholipid was precipitated.

The free fatty acids were then separated from the other cellular neutral lipids by forming a hydrophilic salt. The combined supernatants from the phospholipid precipitation were dried under N_2 and the neutral lipid dissolved in 15 ml petroleum ether; 20 ml 50% ethanol and 0.5 ml 50% KOH were added and the solution stirred for one hr in the cold. The free fatty acids were found in the ethanolic KOH layer. When ^{14}COOH-tripalmitin was subjected to the isolation procedure, 99% of the glyceride was found in the petroleum ether layer. The experiments using labeled triglyceride also indicated that there was no saponification of the triglyceride during the extraction procedure. The fatty acids were then removed from the aqueous phase by acidification to pH 2 with concentrated HCl and extracting three times with 20, 15, and 10 ml ethyl ether. This last partition, coupled with the original aqueous wash procedure of Folch, assures complete separation of the fatty acids from other cellular acids such as lactate and pyruvate.

When the free fatty acid was to be isolated from serum, the serum was acidified with HCl to pH 2 and extracted with 20 volumes chloroform:methanol (2:1). Five volumes of water were then added. After removal of the aqueous phase, the resultant lipid extract was carried through the same procedure as the cellular lipid.

Rat tissues were minced and a weighed aliquot taken for the determination of dry weight. Another weighed aliquot was placed in 20 volumes of warm chloroform:methanol (2:1) and subjected to the same procedures as described for the cellular lipid extract.

The efficiency of the extraction procedure for fatty acids was ascertained by adding ^{14}C-labeled stearic acid to the total lipid extract at the beginning of the procedure. Typically, less than 3% of the free fatty acids are lost in the acetone precipitate, 2-3% are lost in the petroleum ether fraction, and 3-5% are not removed from the aqueous layer. Recoveries range from 85-95% of the original free fatty acid. After the free fatty acids were isolated, they were quantitated by the colorimetric method of Duncombe [15]. This method involves making the cupric salt of the fatty acid and then assaying the copper using diethyl-dithiocarbamate. The possibility that the isolation procedure would interfere with the colorimetric method was assessed by adding a known amount of stearic acid to the cellular lipid extract at the beginning of the procedure. Ninety-eight percent of the stearic acid was recovered in colorimetric determination.

Quantitation of Protein, Glucose and Triglyceride

Protein was measured by the method of Lowry et al.[16] and glucose was quantitated enzymatically by the glucose oxidase procedure (Glucostat – Worthington Biochemicals, Freehold, New Jersey). Triglycerides were measured by the method of van Handel and Zilversmit [17].

Isotopic Studies

Sodium-1-^{14}C acetate, U-^{14}C-glucose, ^{14}COOH-tripalmitin and sodium-1-^{14}C-palmitate were obtained from the New England Nuclear Corp., Boston, Mass., and the tripalmitin and palmitic acid were purified by thin-layer chromatography. Isotopic dilution experiments using these isotopes to determine the source of the cellular free fatty acid were conducted in the following manner: Precursor of known specific activity was added to the medium at the time of subcultivation, the glucose and acetate as aqueous solutions and the palmitate and tripalmitin as emulsions. The specific activity of the cellular free fatty acid at the end of the cultivation time was then determined and compared to that of the precursor used. Radioactivity was measured in a Packard Tri-Carb scintillation spectrometer which was equipped with an external standard. The lipid samples were dried under a stream of N_2 and then dissolved in 15 ml of Bray's solution. [18]. Aqueous samples in less than 1 ml amounts were added directly to 15 ml Bray's solution. Samples were counted long enough to reduce the counting error to 1%. When necessary, they were corrected for quenching, using the external standard. In one experiment, radioactivity of lipids on a thin-layer chromatography plate was assayed using a Packard radioactive scanning unit. The Geiger tube had a linear response, and the relative amounts of activity in each lipid were proportional to the area of each peak recorded graphically.

For assay of lipid biosynthesis, cells were harvested and suspended in a buffered balanced salt solution (approximately 10^7 cells/ml) containing sodium 1-^{14}C-acetate (New England Nuclear Corp., Boston, Mass.) of known specific activity as the sole carbon source. The cell suspension was shaken in a water bath at 37°C and at intervals samples were removed and the cells washed in cold BSS. Lipid was extracted from the cells and subfractionated by TLC according to methods described above. Radioactivity in the various lipid fractions was determined without elution from the silicic acid by the method of Snyder and Stephens [19].

RESULTS AND DISCUSSION

The lipid spectra of early and late passage WI-38 cells are presented in Table I. While there is an increase in the total lipid content of late passage cells, the neutral lipid/phospholipid ratio is the same in both types of cells and resembles that found in rapidly dividing and in stationary cells [7]. The increase in lipid in the late passage cells is significant when calculated on both a dry weight and a cellular basis ($p < .025$). The only significant differences found between specific lipid components are in the phospholipid fraction, the older cells showing significant decreases in the amounts of phosphatidyl ethanolamine ($p < .025$) and phosphatidyl inositol ($p < .025$) and a significant increase in the amount of lecithin ($p < .005$).

The fatty acids of the neutral lipids and phospholipids of early and late passage cells are similar (Table II).

The FFA contents in cultured cells and in several rat tissues are shown in Table III. The data are expressed as μmoles per mg dry weight. The values obtained by this method for the rat liver compare favorably to those reported by Ontko [20] and others [21,22]. It can be seen that the various tissues and cultured cells vary greatly in

Table I. Lipids of Early and Late Passage
WI-38 Cells (%)

	Early Passage	Late Passage
Total lipid (mg/100 mg dry wt)	19 ± 1.5*	25 ± 2.6
Neutral lipid (NL), Total	30 ± 2.2	32 ± 2.5
Percent of Total NL		
Cholesteryl ester	9.3 ± 2.6	11 ± 1.4
Triglyceride	11 ± 1.9	14 ± 1.7
Free fatty acid	29 ± 1.9	32 ± 4.1
Diglyceride	11 ± 2.6	7.7 ± 0.9
Cholesterol	32 ± 1.7	30 ± 2.2
Monoglyceride	7.1 ± 1.3	10 ± 4.4
Phospholipid (PL), Total	69 ± 2.2	68 ± 2.5
Percent of Total PL		
Phosphatidyl ethanolamine	12 ± 1.7	6.9 ± 1.7
Phosphatidyl inositol	15 ± 2.7	8.4 ± 1.7
Phosphatidyl serine	8.0 ± 0.9	8.9 ± 3.4
Lecithin	53 ± 3.7	70 ± 3.8
Sphingomyelin	9.6 ± 1.9	9.6 ± 0.9
Lysolecithin	2.5 ± 0.5	2.5 ± 0.4

*Mean ± S.E. of 8 determinations.

Table II. Fatty Acids of Early and Late Passage WI-38 Cells (%)

Fatty acid	Carbon No.	Neutral lipids		Phospholipids	
		Early Passage (3)*	Late Passage (3)*	Early Passage (5)*	Late Passage (6)*
Myristic	14:0	2.1 ± .57	.41 ± .08	3.2 ± .16	1.8 ± .60
Myristoleic	14:1	trace	trace	trace	trace
Palmitic	16:0	22 ± 2.2	20 ± .91	23 ± 1.8	23 ± 2.0
Palmitoleic	16:1	trace	.40 ± .08	trace	.31 ± .04
Stearic	18:0	17 ± 2.2	19 ± 2.1	17 ± 1.9	20 ± 1.5
Oleic	18:1	33 ± 0.4	31 ± 1.3	32 ± 1.4	30 ± 2.5
Linoleic	18:2	7.1 ± 1.3	10 ± .91	6.1 ± .87	7.5 ± .36
Linolenic	18:3	trace	trace	trace	1.9 ± .20
Arachidonic	20:4	20 ± 3.2	19 ± 1.5	19 ± 2.7	17 ± 1.9

*Number of determinations.

Table III. Free Fatty Acid Contents of
Cultured Cells and Rat Tissues*

Cell or Tissue	μmole free fatty acid (mg dry wt)	μmole free fatty acid (10^8 cells)	μmole free fatty acid (mg lipid)	% total lipid
WI-38	.032	1.60	.149	4.2
WI-38VA13A	.038	0.90	.120	3.4
HeLa	.027	0.61	.166	4.7
Fibroblasts				
Skin	.026	3.40	.125	3.5
Muscle	.073	1.50	.149	4.2
L	.010	0.36	.035	1.0
L5178Y	.010	0.14	.072	2.0
Liver	.008	-	.052	1.5
Muscle	.008	-	.023	0.7
Skin	.015	-	.046	1.3
Lung	.030	-	.180	5.1

*Average of 4 determinations.

the content of free fatty acid. The WI-38 and WI-38VA13A
cells contain .035 μmole/mg dry weight, and this value is
much higher than that contained in the L and L-5178Y cells
or in rat liver, skin and muscle. However, the free fatty
acid contents of the WI-38 and WI-38VA13A cells are not unusual; the HeLa cells, skin fibroblasts and rat lung contain
similar levels of free fatty acid, and the amount in the
muscle fibroblasts is even higher. When the data are expressed as percent total lipid, the WI-38 and WI-38VA13A
cells have approximately 4% free fatty acid. This value
corresponds to values of approximately 5% derived from our
previous studies [7], in which the free fatty acids were

measured by a non-specific acid dichromate oxidation method.
When expressed in this manner, the cells and tissues again
vary in free fatty acid levels. The skin and muscle fibroblast-like lines, WI-38, HeLa, WI-38VA13A cells and the
lung tissue have about 4% free fatty acid, whereas in the L
and L-5178Y cultures and the other rat tissues only approximately 1-2% of the cellular lipid is free fatty acid. It is
also convenient to express the data for the cultured cells
in terms of μmoles of fatty acid/10^8 cells. In this case
the values for L and L-5178Y cells are again clearly lower
than the others, although values obtained for HeLa and
WI-38VA13A cells are lower than those for the more fibroblast-
like cells, perhaps because the cells are smaller.

The Source of Free Fatty Acid in WI-38 Cells

    The extent of biosynthesis of free fatty acids in WI-38
cells was determined by growing the cells in the presence of
U-^{14}C-glucose or sodium 1-^{14}C-acetate. The specific activities of the precursor in the medium and of the free fatty
acid present in the cells after confluency was reached were
determined as described above. The ratios of specific activities are a measure of the percentage of free fatty acid
synthesized from precursor. The results, which are presented in Table IV, indicate that very little free fatty
acid is biosynthesized from either glucose or acetate under
the present growth conditions. The low level of cellular
fatty acid biosynthesis suggests that fatty acid is being
supplied to the cells. Since serum is present in the growth
medium of WI-38 cells, experiments were conducted to determine which serum lipids served as the source of cellular
free fatty acid. Since triglyceride is the most abundant
neutral lipid in serum, the contribution of serum triglyceride to cellular free fatty acid was first assessed.
Tripalmitin-^{14}COOH was added to the medium and the experiment was conducted in the same way as those for glucose and
acetate. In this case the ratios of specific activities are
an indication of the percentage of free fatty acid derived
from uptake of serum triglycerides. The data (Table IV)
show that only 1-2% of the cellular free fatty acid is

Table IV. Percent of WI-38 Free Fatty Acid
Derived from Various Subtrates

	Precursor			
	$U-^{14}C-$ glucose (2)*	$1-^{14}C-$ acetate (2)*	$COOH-^{14}C-$ tripalmitin (2)*	$1-^{14}C-$ palmitate (3)*
Precursor (A)				
Quantity	0.96 mg	0.10 mg	278 μg	0.92†
Specific Activity	245,000	1.118,500	65.8	4907
Cellular FFA (B)				
Quantity	0.217 mg	0.242 mg	362 μg	1.45†
Sp. Act.	1925	2166	1.15	5183
% Biosynthesis				
$\dfrac{\text{Sp. Act. (B)}}{\text{Sp. Act. (A)}}$	0.85	0.18	1.75	103

*Number of experiments
† μmole

derived from serum triglyceride. The results of these experiments thus indicate that serum triglyceride is not the
source of cellular free fatty acid.

The contribution of serum free fatty acid to the cellular pools was now measured. This was accomplished through
an isotopic dilution experiment similar to the others using
$1-^{14}C$-palmitate. The results, shown in Table IV, are calculated on the basis of the free fatty acid in the medium
at both the beginning and the end of the experiment. This
was done because it was noted that the specific activity of
the free fatty acid in the medium dropped during the course
of the experiments; the radioactivity of the free fatty

acid fraction decreased, but the actual amount of free fatty
acid in the medium remained constant. We have found that
hydrolysis of the serum triglyceride replenishes the free
fatty acid during culture and that this hydrolysis accounts
for the decrease in specific activity of the free fatty acid
fraction during the course of the experiment.

The results summarized in Table IV show a close correlation between the specific activities of the free fatty
acid in the cells and in the medium at the end of the experiment. These findings suggest that the cellular free fatty
acid is derived from the serum free fatty acid, but that the
cellular pool is in rapid equilibrium with the medium. If
the intracellular free fatty acid pool were static, its specific activity would be expected to reflect an average of
the medium specific activity at the beginning and end of the
experiment.

Effect of Serum on Free Fatty Acid Levels
of Cultured Cells

Since it had been established that the free fatty acid
level of WI-38 cells was consistent and that the fatty acid
was derived from the serum free fatty acid, experiments were
initiated to compare WI-38 with one of the cell cultures
with lower levels of free fatty acid in an effort to determine what factors influence cellular free fatty acid levels.
The L cell was chosen because much of the work reported on
the lipids of cultured cells has been derived from this line.
Since the L cells in the previous study had been cultured in
the presence of fetal calf rather than calf serum, and since
fetal calf serum contains much less lipid than calf serum,
(its cholesterol content is one-fourth, for example), seemed
possible that the difference in cellular free fatty acid
levels might be due to a difference in the fatty acid contents of the two sera. Therefore, cultures of WI-38 cells
were grown in fetal calf serum for 1-2 months and L cells
(monolayers) were cultured on calf serum for an equal length
of time. The free fatty acid contents of these cultures
were analyzed and compared with those found in WI-38 and

L cells grown in calf and fetal calf sera, respectively.
The data obtained are shown in Table V. It is evident that
the type of serum used in the growth medium does not affect
the free fatty acid level found in each cell.

The possibility that conditions of cultivation might
affect FFA content was also considered. We found that L
cells grown in monolayer or suspension culture had FFA contents (μmoles/mg protein) of 0.024 and 0.023, respectively.
The data suggest that the difference between FFA levels in
L and WI-38 cells cannot be attributed to a difference in
the methods of culture used.

Another difference between the WI-38 and L cells is
that cells harvested from the WI-38 cultures have reached
confluency and are not rapidly dividing, whereas the L cells,
because of the lack of contact inhibition, are actively proliferating at the time of harvest. Therefore, it seemed
possible that the WI-38 cells might have a lower free fatty
acid content during the early days of culture when they are
proliferating rapidly.

The FFA content of WI-38 cells (μmoles/mg protein) at
25%, 66% and 100% confluency is 0.076, 0.054 and 0.051, respectively. Our data indicate that cultured cells and

Table V.   Free Fatty Acids of WI-38 and L Cells
Grown on Calf and Fetal Calf Sera*

Cell	Type of serum	μmoles FFA (mg protein)	μmoles FFA (10^8 cells)
WI-38	Calf	.106	2.10
	Fetal calf	.103	1.90
L	Calf	.023	0.57
	Fetal calf	.025	0.57

*Average of 4 determinations.

tissues can vary greatly in their content of free fatty
acid. WI-38 cells have higher free fatty acid levels than
do cell lines, such as L and L-5178Y, and tissues, such as
liver, skin and muscle. However, WI-38 and WI-38VA13A cells
are not unusual, and other cultured cells such as HeLa and
certain fibroblast-like strains have been shown to have similar free fatty acid levels. The results of the isotope
studies indicate that under the present conditions of culture, the existing cellular free fatty acid of WI-38 cells
is not biosynthesized de novo, but is derived solely from
the free fatty acid of the serum. This observation may be
interpreted in two ways: that the cells are not able to
synthesize fatty acid, or alternatively, that there is a
feedback inhibition or that a repression mechanism is oper-
ative. Bailey [23] has shown that L cells can synthesize
fatty acid, but that synthesis is inhibited when the cells
are grown in the presence of a serum.

The Source of Cellular Lipid in WI-38 Cells

These studies led us to investigate the source of the
total cellular lipid. Initially, the percentage of cellular
lipid arising from de novo synthesis was assessed using
$U-^{14}C$-glucose or sodium $1-^{14}C$-acetate as precursors. We
found that about 8% of the total lipid was synthesized from
glucose and less than 1% from acetate. Experiments with
$^{32}PO_4$ indicated that all the phospholipid phosphorus of
the cell was derived from the exogenous, labeled phosphate.
Since less than 1% of the phospholipid carbon is derived
from acetate, the data suggest that the simple lipid of the
cell is derived from the serum. Using $^{14}COOH$-tripalmitin
and sodium $1-^{14}C$-palmitate, we studied the contribution of
these substrates to the total cellular lipid. The data are
summarized in Table VI. It is evident that the major source
of cell lipid is the serum free fatty acid.

Comparing values for the cellular lipid to the average
specific activity of the free fatty acid during the growth
period, it appears that 85-90% of the cellular lipid is derived from the free fatty acid in the medium. This figure

Table VI. Percent of WI-38 Cellular Lipid
Derived from Various Substrates

	Precursor			
	$U-^{14}C-$ glucose (2)*	$1-^{14}C-$ acetate (2)*	$COOH-^{14}C-$ tripalmitin (2)*	$1-^{14}C-$ palmitate (3)*
Precursor (A)				
Quantity (μg)	830	100	278	271
Specific Activity†	300	857	65.8	22.8
Cellular lipid (B)				
Quantity (μg)	2950	3100	7400	6500
Sp. Act.†	23	5.8	1.5	19.4
% Biosynthesis				
Sp. Act. (B) / Sp. Act. (A)	7.8	0.7	2.3	85

*Number of experiments
†cpm/μg

is close to what one would expect since 7% of the total lipid is derived from glucose and another 10% of the lipid is
sterol which would not be significantly labeled. The results of this experiment, when coupled with the observation
that neither triglyceride nor de novo biosynthesis contri-
butes to cellular lipid, indicate that free fatty acid is
the apparent source of all of the non-sterol lipid of WI-38
cells. The data also suggest that under normal conditions
of culture the cells take up free fatty acid from the medium
and assemble from it the glycerides and phospholipids needed
for cell growth.

We have found that hydrolysis of triglyceride occurs
during the culture period and thus replenishes the free
fatty acid pool. Experiments using labeled tripalmitin
showed that a loss of 2% of triglyceride activity is sufficient to account for all of the fatty acid produced.

The observation that free fatty acid is the primary
source of lipid in WI-38 cells is consistent with the experiments of Mackenzie et al. [24] and also with in vivo
studies by Shapiro [25]. Shapiro has recently demonstrated
that in the intact animal, plasma-free fatty acid, although
it comprises a small proportion of the total plasma lipid,
has a very short half-life. Moreover, he has demonstrated
that although the liver and adipose tissue utilize mainly
triglycerides, the free fatty acid is the primary source of
energy and lipid for all of the other peripheral tissues.
There are several possible mechanisms to explain the hydrolysis of serum triglyceride observed during culture. It
could be mediated by a cellular or a serum enzyme, or simply
be caused by the medium being maintained under slightly alkaline conditions for 7 days at $37^\circ C$. The data suggest that
the primary factor may be an enzyme present in the serum.

Regardless of the mechanism involved, this hydrolysis
of triglycerides could explain the apparent discrepancy between the data obtained in the present study (indicating
that fatty acid is the source of cellular lipid) and the
experiments of Bailey et al. [6], which suggested that triglyceride was the source of cellular lipid. Since Bailey
reported no data for free fatty acid content, it is possible
that the triglyceride was hydrolyzed and entered the cells
as free fatty acid. Bailey used very high cell densities
in the cultures; thus, fatty acid would be used fast enough
for the triglyceride to show a rapid depletion. He also
noted that after triglycerides were completely depleted,
phospholipids were utilized. Again, it is not clear from
his data whether they entered the cells intact.

Lipids of Transformed Cells

The lipid composition of WI-38 and WI-38VA13A cells is given in Table VII. The results for the WI-38 are comparable to those obtained in the previous study [7]. The total lipid content of WI-38VA13A cells is similar to that of WI-38. There is, however, a significant increase in the percentage of neutral lipid present and a concomitant decrease in phospholipid content in the transformed cells (p< .005). A comparison of the actual amounts of neutral lipid and phospholipid present (expressed as mg/100 mg dry weight) suggests that the alteration in distribution is due primarily to a decrease in the amount of phospholipid in the transformed cells. There seems to be no significant difference between the neutral lipid spectra of the normal and transformed cells. Cholesterol and triglycerides are the predominant neutral lipids in both cells, and there are small amounts of cholesteryl ester and mono- and diglycerides.

A comparison of the phospholipids present in WI-38 and WI-38VA13A cells shows lecithin to be predominant. There are also appreciable amounts of sphingomyelin, phosphatidyl ethanolamine and phosphatidyl serine. The content of phosphatidyl inositol is rather large for a non-neural tissue. Plasmalogens and phosphatidic acid were not determined, but they comprise less than 5% of the total phospholipid phosphorus. There are no significant differences between the phospholipid spectra of the two cell types.

The next step in the studies was determination of the fatty acid composition of the WI-38 and transformed cells. The data are presented in Table VIII. The predominant fatty acids found in the neutral lipids of WI-38 were palmitic (16:0) and oleic (18:1); stearic, linoleic and arachidonic acids were also present in appreciable amounts. In comparing these to the fatty acids of the neutral lipids of the transformed cells, we found a significant decrease in the amount of arachidonic acid present in the transformed cells (p < .01) with a concomitant increase in the content of oleic acid (p< .01). The fatty acid spectrum of the phospholipids

Table VII. Lipids of WI-38 and WI-38VA13A Cells (%)

	WI-38	WI-38VA13A
Total lipid (mg/100 mg dry wt)	21 ± 2.3*	18 ± 2.1
Neutral lipid (NL), Total	29 ± 2.3$^{(13)}$†	41 ± 0.9$^{(7)}$
Percent of Total NL		
Cholesteryl ester	5.0 ± 2.1$^{(4)}$	4.0 ± 2.1$^{(6)}$
Triglyceride	27 ± 3.7	25 ± 5.3
Free fatty acid	21 ± 2.9	26 ± 4.2
Diglyceride	6.1 ± 2.5	2.7 ± 1.7
Cholesterol	35 ± 8.7	35 ± 5.7
Monoglyceride	5.2 ± 2.6	6.2 ± 1.3
Phospholipid, (PL), Total	71 ± 2.3$^{(13)}$	59 ± 2.4$^{(7)}$
Percent of Total PL		
Phosphatidyl ethanolamine	12 ± 2.2$^{(8)}$	13 ± 4.2$^{(6)}$
Phosphatidyl inositol	13 ± 3.0	10 ± 0.9
Phosphatidyl serine	12 ± 3.4	4.2 ± 1.3
Lecithin	57 ± 4.6	57 ± 4.0
Sphingomyelin	7.4 ± 0.7	13 ± 2.4
Lysolecithin	2.9 ± 0.3	2.0 ± 0.5

* Mean ± S.E.
†( ) Number of determinations.

Table VIII. Fatty Acids of WI-38 and WI-38VA13A Cells

Fatty acid	Carbon No.	Neutral lipids		Phospholipids	
		WI-38 (6)*	WI-38VA13A (3)*	WI-38 (11)*	WI-38VA13A (5)*
Myristic	14:0	1.3 ± .44	1.2 ± .10	2.1 ± .41	2.3 ± .12
Myristoleic	14:1	trace	trace	trace	trace
Palmitic	16:0	21 ± 1.1	25 ± 1.8	23 ± 1.3	25 ± 1.3
Palmitoleic	16:1	.40 ± .08	trace	.35 ± .04	trace
Stearic	18:0	18 ± 1.4	14 ± 2.0	19 ± 1.2	16 ± 1.3
Oleic	18:1	32 ± .87	42 ± 2.5	31 ± 1.5	36 ± 1.7
Linoleic	18:2	8.6 ± 1.0	11 ± 2.5	6.9 ± .36	9.2 ± 1.2
Linolenic	18:3	trace	trace	1.9 ± .20	trace
Arachidonic	20:4	19 ± 1.6	5.5 ± 2.1	18 ± 1.6	12 ± 2.1

*Number of determinations.

of WI-38 is similar to that of the neutral lipids. In comparing the fatty acids of the phospholipids of the normal
and transformed cells, there is again a significant decrease
in arachidonic acid ($p < .05$) in the transformed cells. There
are several possible explanations for the decreased arachidonic acid levels in the transformed cells. Harary et al.
[26] have reported that newly explanted heart cells lose
their ability to convert linoleic acid to arachidonic acid
after periods in culture; and Geyer et al. [27] found that
the established cell lines HeLa and L cannot synthesize
arachidonic acid and contain it only when grown in the presence of serum. Thus, the lower arachidonic acid content of
the WI-38VA13A cells may be a reflection of the fact that
they have been maintained in culture for a longer time than
have the WI-38 cells and are losing their ability to synthesize this fatty acid. Alternatively, the difference may reflect different intrinsic rates of uptake and utilization of
highly unsaturated fatty acid in the two cell types. It is
interesting that there is a higher arachidonic acid content
in the phospholipids than in the neutral lipids of the transformed cells. This could suggest a preferential utilization
of highly unsaturated fatty acids for membrane structures.
It is also noteworthy that the decrease in arachidonic acid
in the transformed cells is compensated for by an increase
in another unsaturated fatty acid, so that the ratio of saturated to unsaturated acids remains relatively constant.

The synthesis of lipids from $1\text{-}^{14}C$-acetate in the absence of serum by a "resting cell" system was measured. The
cells were found to be capable of synthesizing all of the
lipid classes assayed. In WI-38 cells, after 75 min, about
$2.5\,\mu$moles of ^{14}C-acetate per 10^8 cells were incorporated
into all neutral lipid classes. The incorporation of ^{14}C-
acetate into phospholipid was 5-fold greater. In the WI-
38VA13A cells the results were similar, with the notable exception that the amount of acetate incorporated into cholesterol was almost as high as into phospholipid.

The significance of the observed elevation in rate of
cholesterol biosynthesis in the WI-38VA13A cells is unclear.
Siperstein et al. [28] have presented data suggesting that

certain hepatomas lack feedback mechanisms involved in regulation of cholesterol biosynthesis. It is unlikely, however, that the elevation in rate noted in the present experiments represents a release of the control of cholesterol
synthesis, because the rates observed in both cells are
still far lower than those necessary for cell cholesterol
biosynthesis. Moreover, since the transformed cell is
better able to proliferate, one would not expect it to lose
the regulation of its metabolism.

The similarity of the lipids noted in this study between a diploid cell line and a transformed cell line is
in contrast to reports in the literature citing differences
in phosphatide [29], fatty acid [30,31] and sterol [32] contents between normal and malignant tissues in vivo. Our results do not parallel Gore and Popjak's hypothesis [33] that
neoplastic cells are unable to synthesize cholesterol. It
is possible that since the data obtained in this study represent a precise comparison between an altered cell line and
its known progenitor, none of the previously reported lipid
differences are significant to the malignant process. Alternatively, the differences between these two cell lines
may not be analogous to the differences between normal
and malignant cells in vivo.

SUMMARY

(1) The lipid spectra of early and late passage WI-38
cells are similar, but the late passage cells contain 33%
more lipid.

(2) The fatty acid spectra of the cellular lipids of
early and late passage WI-38 cells are similar.

(3) The WI-38 line of human diploid cells has a re-
markably high content of free fatty acid (4% of the total
lipid).

(4) The cellular free fatty acid of WI-38 cells is
derived from the serum free fatty acid.

(5) Most of the cellular lipid of WI-38 cells is derived from serum free fatty acid.

(6) The total lipid content (mg/100 mg dry wt) of WI-38 and WI-38VA13A cells is similar; however, the transformed cells contain significantly more neutral lipid.

(7) The oleic and linoleic acid contents of WI-38VA13A cells are higher and the arachidonic acid content lower than that of WI-38 cells.

REFERENCES

1. H.E. Swim, "Microbiological aspects of tissue culture," Ann. Rev. Microbiol., 13:141, 1959.

2. J.M. Bailey, "Lipid metabolism of cultured cells. VI. Lipid biosynthesis in serum and synthetic growth medium," Biochim. Biophys. Acta, 125:226, 1966.

3. R.P. Geyer and J.M. Neimark, "Triglyceride utilization by human HeLa and conjunctive cells in tissue culture," Am. J. Clin. Nutr., 7:86, 1959.

4. M.S. Moskowitz, "Fatty acid-induced steatosis in monolayer cell cultures," in: G.H. Rothblat and D. Kritchevsky, Eds., Lipid Metabolism in Tissue Culture Cells, Wistar Inst. Symposium Monograph No. 6. Philadelphia, Wistar Press, 1967, p. 63.

5. G.H. Rothblat, R. Hartzell, H. Mialhe, and D. Kritchevsky, "Cholesterol metabolism in tissue culture cells," in: G.H. Rothblat and D. Kritchevsky, Eds., Lipid Metabolism in Tissue Culture Cells, Wistar Inst. Symposium Monograph No. 6. Philadelphia, Wistar Press, 1967, p. 129.

6. J.M. Bailey, "Lipid metabolism in cultured cells. I. Factors affecting cholesterol uptake," Proc. Soc. Exptl. Biol. Med., 107:30, 1961.

7. D. Kritchevsky and B.V. Howard, "The lipids of human diploid cell strain WI-38," Ann. Med. exp. Fenn., 44:343, 1966.

8. H. Koprowski, J.A. Ponten, F. Jensen, R.G. Ravdin, P. Moorhead, and E. Saksela, "Transformation of cultures of human tissue infected with Simian Virus SV$_{40}$," J. Cell. Comp. Physiol., 59:281, 1962.

9. V.J. Cristofalo and D. Kritchevsky,"Respiration and glycolysis in the human diploid cell strain WI-38," J. Cell.
   Physiol., 67:125, 1966.

10. J.S. Amenta, "A rapid chemical method for quantification
    of lipids separated by thin layer chromatography,"
    J. Lipid Res., 5:270, 1964.

11. C.H. Fiske and Y. Subbarow, "The colorimetric determina-
    tion of phosphorus," J. Biol. Chem., 66:375, 1925.

12. A.T. James, "Qualitative and quantitative determination
    of the fatty acids by gas-liquid chromatography," Meth.
    Biochem. Anal., 8:1, 1960.

13. J. Folch, M. Lees, G.H.S. Stanley, "A simple method for
    the isolation and purification of total lipids from
    animal tissues," J. Biol. Chem., 226:497, 1957.

14. W.R. Bloor, "The oxidative determination of phospholipid
    (lecithin and cephalin) in blood and tissues," J. Biol.
    Chem., 82:273, 1929.

15. W.G. Duncombe, "The colorimetric micro-determination of
    long-chain fatty acids," Biochem. J., 88:7, 1963.

16. O.H. Lowry, N.J. Rosebrough, A.L. Farr, and R.J. Randall,
    "Protein measurement with the Folin phenol reagent,"
    J. Biol. Chem., 193:265, 1951.

17. E. van Handel and D.B. Zilversmit, "Micromethod for the
    direct determination of serum triglycerides," J. Lab.
    Clin. Med., 50:152, 1957.

18. D.L. Trout, E.H. Estes, Jr., and S.J. Freidberg, "Titra-
    tion of free fatty acids in plasma: A study of current
    methods and a new modification," J. Lipid Res., 1:199,
    1960.

19. F. Snyder and N. Stephens, "Quantitative carbon-14 and
    tritium assay of thin-layer chromatography plates, " Anal.
    Biochem., 4:128, 1962.

20. J.A. Ontko, "Chylomicron free fatty acid and ketone body
    metabolism of isolated liver cells and liver homogenates,"
    Biochim. Biophys. Acta, 137:13, 1967.

21. A.A. Stein, E. Opalka, and I. Rosenblum, "Hepatic lipids
    in tumor-bearing (glioma) mice," Cancer Res., 25:957, 1965.

22. D. Sgoutas, "The lipids in normal chicken liver," Can.
    J. Biochem., 44:763, 1966.

23. J.M. Bailey, "Cellular lipid nutrition and lipid trans-
    port," in: G.H. Rothblat and D. Kritchevsky, Eds., Lipid
    Metabolism in Tissue Culture Cells, Wistar Inst. Symp.
    Monograph No. 6. Philadelphia, Wistar Press, 1967, p. 85.
24. C.G. Mackenzie, J.G. Mackenzie, and O.K. Reiss, "Regula-
    tion of cell lipid metabolism and accumulation. V. Quan-
    titative and structural aspects of triglyceride accumula-
    tion stimulated by lipogenic substances," in: G.H.
    Rothblat and D. Kritchevsky, Eds., Lipid Metabolism in
    Tissue Culture Cells, Wistar Inst. Symp. Monograph No. 6.
    Philadelphia, Wistar Press, 1967, p. 63.
25. B. Shapiro, "Biochemistry of triglycerides," in: G.
    Schettler, Ed., Lipids and Lipidosis. New York, Springer-
    Verlag, Inc., 1967, p. 40.
26. I. Harary, L.E. Gerschenson, D.F. Haggerty, W. Desmond,
    and J.F. Mead, "Fatty acid metabolism and function in
    cultured heart and HeLa cells," in: G.H. Rothblat and
    D. Kritchevsky, Eds., Lipid Metabolism in Tissue Culture
    Cells, Wistar Inst. Symp. Monograph No. 6. Philadelphia,
    Wistar Press, 1967, p. 17.
27. R.P. Geyer, A. Bennett, and A. Rohr, "Fatty acids of the
    triglycerides and phospholipids of HeLa cells and strain
    L fibroblasts," J. Lipid Res., 3:80, 1962.
28. M.D. Siperstein, V.M. Fagan, and H.P. Morris, "Further
    studies on the deletion of the cholesterol feedback
    system in hepatomas," Cancer Res., 26:7, 1966.
29. C. Carruthers, and A. Heining, "Phosphatides in mouse
    epidermis undergoing normal and abnormal growth changes,"
    Cancer Res., 24:485, 1964.
30. B. Gerstl, R.B. Hayman, P. Ramorino, M.G. Tavaststjerna,
    "Lipids of malignant tumors," Am. J. Clin. Pathol.,
    43:314, 1965.
31. C. Carruthers, "The fatty acid composition of the phos-
    phatides of normal and malignant epidermis," Cancer Res.,
    27:1, 1967.
32. J. Kawanami, T. Tsuji, and H. Otsuka, "Lipids of cancer
    tissues. I. Lipid composition of Shinogi Carcinoma 115
    and Nakahara-Fukuoka Sarcoma," J. Biochem. (Tokyo),
    59:151, 1966.
33. I.Y. Gore and G. Popjak, "Sterol biosynthesis in neoplas-
    tic cells: utilization of ^{14}C-acetate and 2-^{14}C-mevalo-
    nate," Biochem. J., 84:93, 1962.

METABOLIC ASPECTS OF AGING IN DIPLOID HUMAN CELLS*

Vincent J. Cristofalo†

The Wistar Institute of Anatomy and Biology
Philadelphia, Pennsylvania

Aging may reflect, in part, the outcome of environmental stresses on cells and tissues; a question of major
interest, however, is whether a mechanism independent of
the environment exists at the cellular level and operates
in such a manner that senescence and death are the pro-
grammed destiny of normal mammalian cells and tissues. A
model system which allows an approach to some aspects of
this question is provided by the diploid human cell lines
[1,2]. During serial subcultivation these cells retain
many of the characteristics of normal cells in situ, such
as a stable diploid karyotype and sex chromatin in the
interphase nuclei of female cells. In addition, it is
now well established that these normal cells will proliferate in culture for varying, but finite periods of

*Supported, in part, by U.S. Public Health Service Research
Grant RO1-HD 02721 from the National Institute of Child
Health and Human Development and Pa. Dept. of Health Con-
tract 69-593-1,ME-561 from the Commonwealth of Pennsylvania.
†Associate Professor of Biochemistry, Division of Animal
Biology, School of Veterinary Medicine, University of
Pennsylvania, Philadelphia, Pennsylvania.

time; and that following a period of rapid and vigorous proliferation, the growth of the population slows down, the cells become granular, debris accumulates, and ultimately, the culture degenerates.

Detailed experiments have shown that cultures of fetal human lung cells have a doubling potential of between 40 and 60 generations. Hayflick and Moorhead [1] presented evidence that this cellular deterioration was not a direct effect of nutritional deficiencies, microcontaminants, or the elaboration of toxic products by the cells, and interpreted this phenomenon as aging at the cellular level. Although, thus far, the relationship between aging in vitro and aging in vivo has not been clearly delineated, the phenomenon of senescence in human cell cultures does appear to make them a very useful model system for studying the cellular mechanism of aging in vivo.

In addition, these cells, which have a normal human karyotype and display non-malignant growth in vivo, can be transformed by SV40 virus into cultures which are mixoploid, which show malignant-type growth in vivo and which have an indefinite life span [3]. Thus, we have at our disposal young, normal cells which undergo aging (in terms of their ability to proliferate) and sister cultures of transformed cells, which have an indefinite life span.

In order to elucidate the mechanism underlying these differences, we have been comparing some aspects of the metabolism of these cells. The results of investigations into three areas of cellular metabolism comprise the basis for this report.

RESULTS

I. Glucose Metabolism

One of our first observations with the diploid human
cells was that their rate of proliferation directly paralleled
their rate of glucose utilization [4,5]. Since the rate
of proliferation is a measure of the vigor or age of the
population, a study of the characteristics of glucose
metabolism seemed to be worthwhile.

Figure 1 summarizes several pathways of glucose metabolism. Glucose occupies a central position in cellular
metabolism and the various transformations of glucose en-
compass a wide variety of functions necessary to the growth,
multiplication, and integrity of the cell. The interconver-
sions of glucose provide: a) energy through glycolysis and
respiration; b) building blocks for the various macromolecules synthesized by the cell, including the ribose and
deoxyribose elements of the nucleic acids; and c) the re-
ducing power, principally as NADPH, necessary for the synthesis of a wide variety of biologically important compounds.
Thus far, we have studied respiration and glycolysis in
intact cells, as well as some of the key enzymes involved
in glucose metabolism, both in the glycolytic pathway and
in the oxidative and nonoxidative limbs of the pentose phosphate shunt.

For all of these studies we have used diploid human
cell line WI-38 and the permanently proliferating cell
line WI-38 VA13, which was derived from WI-38 by SV40 virus-
transformation. Details of the method of subcultivation

have been described in previous publications [4,6].
In general, the cells were grown in 2-liter Povitzky
bottles. Eagle's medium (BME) containing twice the concentration of amino acids and vitamins, prepared in
Earle's balanced salt solution and supplemented with 10%
calf serum was used routinely [7].

For metabolic studies, cells which were approaching
the end of the log phase of growth (2/3-3/4 confluency)
were removed from the glass surface by trypsinization.
The cells were concentrated by centrifugation at 500 X g
for three min at 4°C, washed 3 times with a phosphate-
buffered balanced salt solution and used immediately for
the experiments. For all but the respiratory studies,
one-half of the medium was replaced with fresh medium 24
hr before harvesting. Standard manometric techniques
were used for studies of respiration [8]. Details of
these methods have also been described elsewhere [6].
The rationale for both the choice of the enzymes of glucose metabolism that we studied and the methods of measurement we used, is shown by a consideration of Figure 1.
We measured hexokinase activity since this is the first
enzyme involved in glucose utilization. The product of
hexokinase reaction, glucose-6-phosphate, represents a
branch-point in glucose metabolism, so we compared two of
the enzymes which compete for glucose-6-phosphate, phosphoglucose isomerase and glucose-6-phosphate dehydrogenase.
We also assayed 6-phosphogluconate dehydrogenase. The
product of the phosphoglucose isomerase reaction, fructose-
6-phosphate, also represents a branch-point in glucose
metabolism interacting either with the enzymes of the non-
oxidative limb of the hexosemonophosphate shunt pathway,

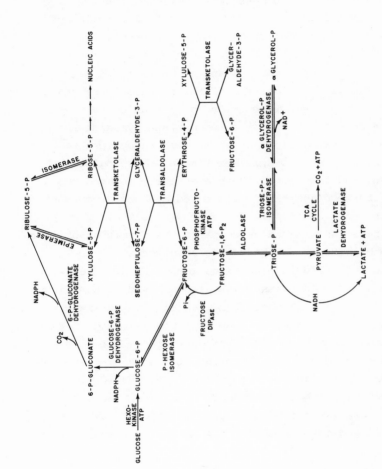

Fig. 1. Pathways of glucose metabolism.

transaldolase and transketolase, or with the enzyme
phosphofructokinase, which, together with fructose diphosphatase, is considered to constitute the major control
point in glycolysis; we measured these four interrelated
enzymes. Finally, we included the terminal reaction of
glycolysis, lactate dehydrogenase. In general, the
methods of enzyme analysis were adapted from those described by Shonk and Boxer [9] and by Novello and McLean
[10]. The maximal velocities of the reaction were measured.
by coupling the specific enzymes to be studied to the
oxidation or reduction of the appropriate pyridine nucleotides and following the changes in absorbancy spectro-
photometrically at 340 mμ. Hexokinase, phosphoglucose-
isomerase, and fructose diphosphatase were assayed by
coupling these reactions to those mediated by glucose-6-
phosphate and 6-phosphogluconate dehydrogenase. Phosphofructokinase was assayed by coupling the formation of fructose diphosphate to the reduction of glyceraldehyde-3-
phosphate and following the oxidation of NADH. Transaldolase and transketolase were also assayed by coupling
to this reaction sequence. For transaldolase a mixture
of fructose-6 and erythrose-4-phosphates was used as substrate and for transketolase, ribose-5-phosphate plus an
enzyme preparation from rat spleen [11] which mediated the
production of a mixture of ribulose-5-phosphate, xylulose-
5-phosphate and ribose-5-phosphate was used. Lactate
dehydrogenase was measured in the direction of pyruvate
to lactate and the oxidation of NADH was followed.

The packed cells were suspended in 9 volumes of extraction medium [9] and homogenized in a Potter-Elvejhem
homogenizer. The resulting homogenate was centrifuged at

105,000 X g for 1 hr and the precipitate was discarded.
When fructose diphosphatase was to be assayed, an aliquot
was removed from the crude homogenate and centrifuged at
10,000 X g for 15 min.

All of the enzymes were assayed at room temperature
(23-27°C) in 0.05 M triethanolamine buffer at pH 7.5,
containing .006 M EDTA. The pH, which was checked before
and after each assay, never varied more than -0.3 units
from the starting pH of 7.6. Except for fructose diphosphatase and hexokinase, the total activity of all the
enzymes could be recovered in the 100,000 X g supernatant.
Protein determinations were carried out according to the
method of Lowry et al. [12].

No attempt was made to select optimal conditions for
each enzyme since our real purpose was to compare the activities of these enzymes under the same conditions; however,
for each assay, the velocity of the reaction was always
proportional to the amount of cell homogenate added and
was always linear with respect to the time of incubation.
Details of the method used for the determination of each
enzyme will be published elsewhere.

It is important to note that the activity of enzymes
derived from disrupted cells and assayed under optimal,
or nearly optimal, conditions does not necessarily reflect
their activity in the intact cell. However, the relationship among the activities of a series of enzymes measured
under similar conditions probably reflects the relative
capacities of the individual steps in the various pathways
under consideration. By combining this kind of data with
the results of studies of intact cells,one can obtain a

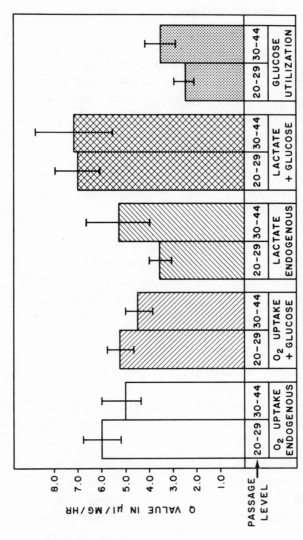

Fig. 2. The influence of passage number on respiration and glycolysis in WI-38 cells. A summary of all the measurements obtained at the different passage levels. The numbers between the base of the bar and the parameter designation show the range of passages that the measurement represents. The figures show mean values ± standard error of the mean (n=9 for passages 20–29 and 10 for passages 30–44).

meaningful profile of the various metabolic pathways.

Figure 2 summarizes the effect of age on the respiration
and glycolysis of intact WI-38 cells. Mean values for cells
at passage levels above and below 30 were compared. Oxygen
uptake with and without glucose, glucose utilization,
and lactate production, both from endogenous reserves
and from glucose, were all equivalent for the two groups.
Although not shown in this figure, quantitatively similar
data have been obtained for the transformed WI-38 VA13
cells and no differences among these three groups of
cells were evident.

From these data we can conclude that the aging process
in WI-38 cells is not accompanied by any changes in their
respiratory or glycolytic capacities. Support for this
conclusion has come from the recent work of Hakami and
and Pious [13] in which they found no age-dependent reduction in cytochrome oxidase activity in senescent human
fibroblasts and no differences between virus-transformed
and non-transformed cells.

Although there are few reports which are precisely
comparable to ours from the point of view of aging, some
studies which attempted to establish the relationship
between metabolic capacity and age have been carried out
with mammalian tissue slices and homogenates. The data
from these studies have varied greatly and the results
have been inconclusive. Reiner [14] studied the effect
of age on the carbohydrate metabolism of rat tissue homogenates and observed a decline only in tissue taken from
rats over 2 years of age. Rafsky et al. [15] studied

age differences in the respiration of guinea pig tissue
homogenates and reported that liver homogenates showed
no change between 8-100 weeks of age, whereas kidney
homogenates showed some decline. Barrows and co-workers
[16] compared the rates of O_2 consumption and anaerobic
glycolysis in liver and kidney slices of rats 12-14 and
24-27 months of age. No differences were found in the
rates of anaerobic glycolysis or respiration of liver,
but here again, some decline was found for kidney.
More recently Gold   et   al. [17] have reported that there
is no age-associated decrease in oxidative phosphorylation
in mitochondria isolated from rat kidney, heart and liver.

The studies discussed above were directly concerned
with aging at the organism or organ level and, as such, are
not really comparable to ours. The net changes that were
observed could reflect the results of either interaction
among the different organ systems or the decline of one
cell type and not another in the same organ. The present studies deal with a single cell type in pure culture
which manifests properties resembling physiological senescence. The fact that this phenomenon is not accompanied
by changes in metabolic capability supports the original
qualitative observations of Hayflick and Moorhead [1]
that the cells entering phase III continue to have a high
rate of metabolic activity despite the very low rate of
mitotic activity.

Table I summarizes the values obtained for the maximal
activities of a number of glycolytic enzymes. Both the
normal WI-38 cells and the transformed cells show a spectrum of enzymatic activity typical of a relatively highly
glycolyzing cell type, i.e., fructose diphosphatase activity
is very low, lactate dehydrogenase and phosphoglucose

Table I. Enzymes of Glucose Metabolism
in Human Cells

Cell type	Passage level	Mean specific activity in $m\mu$ moles/min/mg protein				
		Hexokinase	Phosphoglucose-isomerase	Phospho-fructokinase	Fructose diphosphatase	Lactic dehydrogenase
WI-38	20-46	10. 74 ± 1. 24 (32)	633. 7 ± 72 (32)*	54. 31 ± 3. 65 (20)	4. 24 ± 0. 67 (18)	2170 ± 126 (52)
WI-38 VA13A	----	8. 09 ± 0. 93 (12)	1058. 9 ± 27 (12)*	51. 33 ± 6. 70 (10)	2. 38 ± 0. 23 (10)	2352 ± 156 (13)
WI-38	20-25	9. 93 ± 1. 78 (8)	735. 3 ± 194 (8)*	61. 83 ± 5. 73 (6)	3. 84 ± 0. 34 (5)	2152 ± 173 (8)
WI-38	26-33	13. 99 ± 2. 27 (14)	753. 2 ± 98 (14)	54. 14 ± 5. 77 (8)	5. 90 ± 1. 43 (7)	2200 ± 200 (20)
WI-38	33-46	6. 85 ± 0. 69 (10)	385. 2 ± 40 (10)	47. 02 ± 6. 18 (6)	2. 63 ± 0. 51 (6)	2152 ± 48 (24)

* WI-38 VA13A significantly different from WI-38 at all passage levels $p < .005$

isomerase activities are relatively high, and hexokinase
and phosphofructokinase show relatively low activities
typical of their "pacemaker" function. The total hexokinase
activity agrees closely with the value for glucose utilization in intact cells. The hexokinase activity shown
here represents the specific activity of the non-particulate
fraction; however, for both the normal and transformed cells,
a constant fraction of the hexokinase is bound to the par-
ticulate material of the cells and inclusion of the activity
from this fraction would raise the value for total hexokinase
in each case by about 20 units.

We compared the activities of these enzymes in young,
intermediate, and old cells and in transformed cells.
Although there are some variations, only phosphoglucose
isomerase shows differences that are statistically significant; the transformed cells had an activity two-fold
higher than the normal cells $(p < .005)$. Since the overall
glycolytic rates are the same, this finding is difficult
to interpret; one possibility is that the high activity
in transformed cells reflects a greater production of

fructose-6-phosphate for further transformation through
the non-oxidative limb of the pentose shunt since phosphoglucose isomerase competes with glucose-6-phosphate
dehydrogenase for glucose-6-phosphate. An alternative
possibility is that the high level of phosphoglucose
isomerase represents an adaptive mechanism of the transformed cells to overcome the inhibition of this enzyme
by 6-phosphogluconate which may accumulate as a result
of the high ratio of glucose-6-phosphate dehydrogenase
to 6-phosphogluconate dehydrogenase (Table II) [18].

    The finding that there were no differences in the
activities of the glycolytic enzymes during aging supports
the data obtained from intact cells which shows that
the glycolytic rate does not vary as cell senescence pro-
gresses.

Table II.   Enzymes of Glucose Metabolism
in Human Cells

Cell type	Passage level	Mean specific activity in $m\mu$ moles/min/mg protein			
		Glucose-6-phosphate dehydrogenase	6-phosphogluconate dehydrogenase	Transaldolase	Transaketolase
WI-38	20-46	146. 9 ± 18 (31)	14. 28 ± 1. 3 (32)	41. 30 ± 3. 28 (20)[†]	5. 69 ± 0. 60 (20)
WI-38 VA13A	----	101. 5 ± 14 (12)	8. 96 ± 1. 1 (12)*	15. 75 ± 0. 90 (10)[†]	7. 08 ± 0. 26 (11)
WI-38	20-25	113. 6 ± 22 (8)	17. 28 ± 2. 8 (8)**	43. 38 ± 5. 69 (6)	8. 03 ± 0. 96 (6)[‡]
WI-38	26-33	152. 1 ± 12 (14)	16. 70 ± 1. 9 (14)**	45. 66 ± 5. 87 (8)	4. 61 ± 0. 74 (8)[‡]
WI-38	33-46	163. 8 ± 52 (9)	8. 47 ± 0. 81 (10)**	33. 41 ± 3. 26 (6)	4. 80 ± 0. 89 (6)[‡]

    * WI-38 VA13A significantly different from WI-38 passages 20-33 $p < .01$

    ** Passages 33-46 signifcantly different from the other two groups $p < .005$

    † WI-38 significantly different from WI-38 VA13A $p < .001$

    ‡ Passages 20-25 significantly different from two later passage groups $p < .02$

Table II shows the activities for the enzymes of the
hexose monophosphate shunt. For both cell types, as
with most tissues, glucose-6-phosphate dehydrogenase
activity was higher than 6-phosphogluconate dehydrogenase
activity and transaldolase activity was higher than transketolase. Thus, 6-phosphogluconate dehydrogenase appears
to be rate-limiting for the oxidative pathway while transketolase appears to be the rate-limiting enzyme for the
entire sequence. Glucose-6-phosphate dehydrogenase activity is similar in transformed cells and in normal cells
at all passage levels. However, 6-phosphogluconate dehydrogenase activity is significantly lower in the oldest
passage levels of the normal cells, as compared with the
young and intermediate passage levels. Transketolase
activity also shows a significant decline in the oldest
cell groups and possibly both of these changes reflect
a reduced rate of synthesis of ribose-5-phosphate for ultimate conversion to nucleotides and nucleic acids in the
slowly proliferating older cultures.

On the other hand, if we compare 6-phosphogluconate
dehydrogenase in transformed cells and in the two younger
groups of normal cells, then the activity in the permanently proliferating transformed cells is significantly
lower than that in the normal cells. Transaldolase activity is also significantly reduced in the transformed cells.
One explanation of these observations might be that they
reflect a lower overall contribution of the entire pentose
phosphate shunt pathway in transformed cells. An alternative explanation would be based on a report by Miedema
and Kruse [19] in which they showed that there was a
significant increase in glucose-6-phosphate dehydrogenase
activity in post-confluent, as compared with pre-confluent
diploid cells, while a number of permanently proliferating

cell lines showed no such differences. None of the cultures that we used could be considered post-confluent.
However, the differences we observed may reflect an extension of basic differences in cellular control mechanisms between normal and transformed cells.

As discussed above, the reduced values for phospho-
gluconate dehydrogenase activity may also be related to the
high value of phosphoglucose isomerase activity in the transformed cells. It is known that 6-phosphogluconate inhibits
phosphoglucose isomerase activity [18,20] and the increased activity of this enzyme in transformed cells may
arise as a result of the increase in 6-phosphogluconate
concentration.

2. Cell Size and Nucleic Acid Content

Along with our studies of glucose metabolism, we began a second area of investigation concerned with nucleic
acid metabolism.

For these studies the cells were cultivated as described above. The nucleic acids were extracted and estimated according to the Schneider modification of the
Schmidt-Thannhauser procedure [21]. Table III shows the
average DNA content per 10^6 cells, calculated by regression
lines based on the method of least squares. The value of
7.94 ± 0.55 µg represents the mean value for 30 determinations of cells from all passages. It is comparable to
values determined cytospectrophotometically by Rudkin et al.[22]
for diploid cell DNA ($7.3 \cdot 10^{-6}$ µg/cell) and is slightly
lower than those reported by Tedesco and Mellman [23] using
a method similar to ours for determination of DNA in human
leucocytes and human skin fibroblast cultures.

Table III.   DNA and RNA Content of WI-38 Cells

Passage	DNA Content		RNA Content		RNA/DNA
	μg/10^6 Cells	μg/mg Protein	μg/10^6 Cells	μg/mg Protein†	
19-27	7.83±1.19 (9)	29.8±7.15 (6)	20.4±3.8 (9)	73.5±21.5(6)	2.924±.54 (9)
28-34	7.58± .898(11)	39.6±9.42 (8)	23.8±3.1 (11)	105.0±13.4 (8)	3.262±.303 (11)
35-54	8.45± .887(10)	50.5±18.2 (4)	30.8±4.3 (10)	199.9±44.8 (4)	3.67 ±.408 (4)
19-54*	7.94± .55 (39)				

For these studies, the cells were allowed to proliferate until they reached about one-half confluency. The used medium was then replaced with fresh medium and, after 24 hours, the cells were harvested and the nucleic acids extracted and estimated (Volkin and Cohn, 1954). The figures show the mean ± SE (number of determinations).

* Mean value for all passages.

† Passages 19-27 significantly different from passages 35-54 (p<.01).

Grouping the data into values obtained from young, intermediate, and old passage material, and evaluation of the mean nucleic acid content suggests in each case a trend toward increasing values in older cells.   However, statistical analysis of these data shows that significant differences among groups are evident only for the RNA content per mg protein where there is a significant difference between cultures below passage 27 and those above passage 35 (p<.01).   Regression analysis shows that there is a statistically significant positive association between RNA/mg protein and passage number, as indicated by the correlation coefficient (r=0.73; p<.01).

These findings indicate that some aspects of macromolecular synthesis may occur independently of cell division, and lead to the speculation that diploid human cells in phase III may not have an impaired capability for

protein and RNA synthesis, but rather may be unable either
to carry out DNA synthesis or to accomplish cell division
successfully. This speculation is supported by the
findings of Macieira-Coelho et al. [24], who have shown
by autoradiographic techniques that late passage cultures
of diploid human cells seem to be inhibited in the G1 or
G2 period of the division cycle. Their data indicate that
only a small proportion of phase III cells are synthesi_
zing DNA during any given short period of time. In contrast, RNA synthesis, though reduced in rate, is
occurring in 100% of the phase III cells.

We can postulate that the cell is inhibited in its
ability to divide, but not in its ability to grow, i.e.,
to increase in size. This leads to the conclusion that
phase III cells should be larger than phase II cells.
To determine whether this was so, cells at 4 different
passages were allowed to reach about one-half confluency.
One-half the medium was changed, as described above,
and 24 hr later the cells were harvested and suspended in
a buffered, balanced salt solution. The cells assumed
a spherical shape and the diameters of the cells could be
measured with an ocular micrometer (Figure 3). Each bar
graph represents 100 measurements, and the results show
clearly that the average cell size is significantly increased in older populations. Simons [25] has reported
similar findings obtained in a more extensive study of a
number of cell populations derived from adult human skin.
He has shown that variation in cell size reflects the
changes occurring in aging populations; for example, in
the degenerative phase there is a general broadening of
the frequency of cell diameters. His data also show that

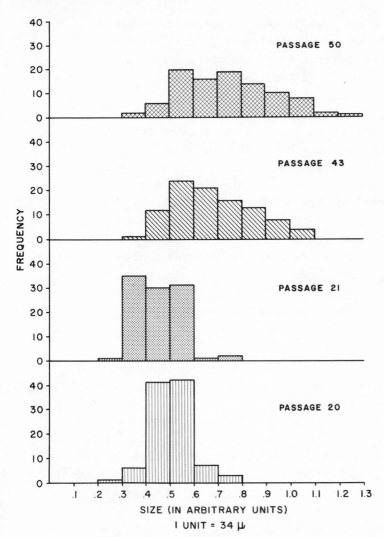

Fig. 3. The influence of passage number on the size of WI-38 cells. The heights of the bars represent the percentage of the cells in each size class. For each passage level 100 cells were measured.

the limited survival of these populations is not a
function of serum specificity, since cell strains cultured in medium containing autologous serum degenerated
as rapidly as cells in medium containing homologous
serum.

There are a number of interpretations for both the
increase in RNA content of older cells and for the increase in cell size. One simple explanation is that
the older cell is capable both qualitatively and quantitatively of all the activities of the young cell, except possibly DNA synthesis or cell division or both.
Presumably, division is inhibited in the G1 phase of the
cell cycle since there is no significant increase of DNA
content per cell. However, the RNA content increases not
only on a cellular basis, but also on a protein basis.
Since protein per cell does not decrease [26], then a
disproportionate synthesis of RNA must occur.

Wulff et al. [27] have investigated the RNA content
of various rat tissues during aging. Their findings showed
that RNA content increased in some tissues, decreased in
others, and in still a third group, remained the same.
Studies of labelled cytidine incorporation indicated that
the changes in RNA content were a function of the changes
in capacity for RNA synthesis. Presumably, age-related
damage to sites and mechanisms for RNA synthesis causes
the production of defective RNA which then produces defective protein. Overproduction of RNA could then be the
result of compensatory increased synthesis due to the absence of the correct product protein.

3. Lysosomal Enzymes

The final area we investigated was the activity of
lysosomal enzymes during aging. These organelles are involved in autolysis resulting from inflammatory processes, as well as in programmed involutional changes such
as the resorption of the tadpoles' tail [28]. Allison
and Paton [29] reported that the lysosomes of WI-38 cells
contain a DNA depolymerase which can cause chromosome
breaks and which can destroy both strands of DNA with a
single hit [30].

We have been measuring the activity of two lysosomal
enzymes, acid phosphatase and β-glucuronidase, during
the aging of WI-38 cells. For these studies the cells
were prepared as described above. The phosphatase was
determined by an adaption of the method of Bessey, Lowry
and Brock [31], which depends on the enzymatic hydrolysis
of p-nitrophenylphosphate. Appropriate aliquots of cell
homogenate were incubated with citrate (0.05 M;pH 5.0)
buffered substrate for 30 min at 37°C. The reaction was
stopped by the addition of alkali and the product of the
reaction, p-nitrophenol, was measured colorimetrically at
410 mµ. β-glucuronidase was measured at pH 4.5 according
to the method of Fishman [32], using phenolphthalein glu-
curonide as substrate.

For these studies, enzyme activities of diploid human
cell strain WI-38 were measured at different passage
levels ranging between 15 and 45. The data obtained were
arbitrarily divided into three groups: young (passages 15-
25), intermediate (passages 25-33), and "senescent" (passages 33-45). The senescent group included cultures with a

decreased proliferation rate and cultures which no
longer grew to confluency. For purposes of comparison
two other cultures were included: (a) human fetal lung
fibroblasts (A-11-L) of undetermined but presumably
diploid karyotype; these were measured before reaching
passage 10 and thus were "younger" than the earliest
WI-38 cultures measured; and (b) a culture of diploid
fibroblasts derived from human adult lung (WI-1006) obtained from a donor whose age at autopsy was 58 [2].
These adult lung fibroblasts have a doubling potential of
only about 20 generations, and in terms of their life span,
they were equivalent to the older cultures of WI-38.
They were studied at passages 13-15.

Figure 4 summarizes the acid phosphatase activity of
these cultures. Cells at passage levels above 35 have a
significantly higher activity than cells of less than 25
passages (p<0.001). The intermediate-age cells show activity intermediate between the young and old cells and
are not significantly different from either. Cultures of
human fetal lung fibroblasts studied between passages 6
and 10 have activities similar to the young WI-38 cultures, while the lung fibroblasts of adult origin show
acid phosphatase activity similar to that of old WI-38 cells.

Superimposed on the bars in figure 4 and representing
the mean acid phosphatase activities are the activities
found for a single series of continuous mother-daughter
subcultivations between passages 22 and 42. These data
also show a rising level of acid phosphatase activity with
an increasing number of subcultivations, indicating that
the increase in the mean value of the activity is not an
artifact of our method of designating cell population age.

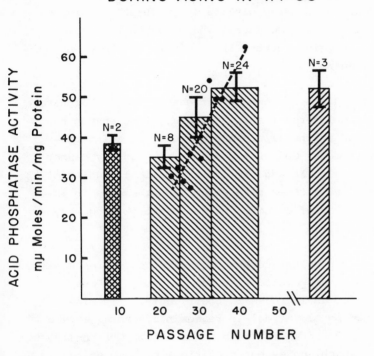

ACID PHOSPHATASE ACTIVITY
DURING AGING IN WI-38

Fig. 4. Acid phosphatase activity during the aging
human diploid cells. Assays were carried out as
described in the text. Mean enzyme activity is
expressed by the heights of the bars and the standard
error of the mean by the brackets. N is the number of
determinations.

⬚ Strain A-11 L   ⬚ Strain WI-38   ⬚ Strain WI-1006

Similar data were obtained for β-glucuronidase activity.

This consistent increase in acid phosphatase and β-glucuronidase activity in WI-38 cells, together with the correlative evidence obtained with adult diploid lung fibroblasts and presumably diploid lung fibroblasts passaged very few times in culture, indicates that a real association may exist between the activity of these enzymes and cellular aging.

Zorzoli [33] has shown an increase in acid phosphatase activity in the livers of aging animals. This enzyme has also been found in the lipofuscin granules of aging tissues as described by Gedigk and Bontke [34] and by Essner and Novikoff [35]. In addition, histochemical studies of young and old rat tissues have shown that there is an increase in activity of a number of dephosphorylating enzymes in the tissue of old rats [36].

Both acid phosphatase and β-glucuronidase are usually considered to be associated with the lysosomes. Possible explanations for an increase in their activity in older cultures would be: 1) a real increase in lysosomal enzyme concentration; 2) an increase in the fragility of the lysosomal membrane which, under our conditions of homogenization, permits more rapid activation of the enzyme, resulting in an increased reaction rate; 3) the possibility, suggested by our studies on the heterogeneity of molecular form and location of acid phosphatase [37] , that the increase in acid phosphatase may not be lysosomal at all, but may occur in some other subcellular fraction. To investigate these three possibilities, we initiated a series of experiments designed to compare both the specific activity and the relative amount

Table IV. The Subcellular Distribution of Acid
Phosphomonoesterase Activity in WI-38 Cells

Passage level	Specific activity*			
	Fraction			
	Nuclear	Lysosomal	Microsomal	Supernatant
17-25	21.33 ± 1.49 (4)	64.07 ± 6.46 (4)	22.20 ± 6.32 (4)	14.68 ± 2.15 (4)[†]
26-35	24.48 ± 2.24 (4)	69.58 ± 6.46 (4)	35.70 ± 6.23 (4)	17.31 ± 3.98 (4)
36-50	27.28 ± 2.91 (9)	89.59 ± 11.2 (9)	41.86 ± 6.90 (9)	21.90 ± 0.72 (9)[†]

* mμ moles/minute/mg protein.

[†] $p < .005$.

The values show the mean ± standard error of the mean
followed by the number of determinations in parentheses.

Table V. The Subcellular Distribution of
β-Glucuronidase Activity in WI-38 Cells

Passage level	Specific activity*			
	Fraction			
	Nuclear	Lysosomal	Microsomal	Supernatant
17-25	11.86 ± 1.37 (4)	42.28 ± 8.58 (4)	12.42 ± 3.12 (4)	5.99 ± 1.08 (4)[†]
26-35	13.92 ± 2.73 (4)	58.84 ± 3.62 (4)	17.71 ± 3.91 (4)	11.67 ± 1.65 (4)
36-50	18.32 ± 1.89 (9)	70.24 ± 9.45 (9)	25.15 ± 3.22 (9)	14.04 ± 1.60 (9)[†]

* μg/hour/mg protein.

[†] $p < 0.01$.

The values show the mean ± the standard error of the mean
followed by the number of determinations in parentheses.

of the activity in the various subcellular fractions
during aging.

For preparation of the various subcellular fractions,
all operations were carried out at or near 4°C. The cells
were suspended in 10^{-3} M phosphate buffer at pH 7.2 and
stirred gently for 10 min. This treatment was followed
by homogenization with a Dounce apparatus using, first, a
loose-fitting, and then a tight-fitting plunger. Microscopic examination of random samples of the homogenate
showed that virtually complete cell breakage resulted from
this treatment. Immediately following the homogenization,
0.5 M sucrose was added to the mixture to give a final sucrose concentration of 0.25 M. The various fractions were
then separated by centrifugation. Four subcellular fractions resulted from this procedure: 1) a nuclear fraction
sedimented at 500 X g (10 min); 2) a lysosomal-mitochondrial
fraction sedimenting at 12,500 X g (20 min); 3) a microsomal
fraction which was sedimented at 105,000 X g (30 min); and
4) the supernatant. Following separation, each fraction was
treated with Triton X-100 (1% final concentration), and the
enzymatic activity was then assayed.

The subcellular distribution of acid phosphatase activity during aging is shown in Table IV. All of the fractions show an increase with activity in aging and the increase in the lysosomal fraction is sufficient to account
for the increase noted in the whole homogenates. Statistical analysis of the data, however, shows that the most
pronounced increase in activity occurs in the supernatant
fraction ($p < .005$).

Similar analysis of the β-glucuronidase activity (Table V) gives similar results, with the supernatant fraction showing a 2-fold difference between the youngest and the oldest groups (p<.01).

Since protein distribution per fraction does not shift during aging, the data show a disproportionate quantity of these two enzymes in the non-particulate fraction of senescent cells and may indicate an increase in the mobility of lysosomal enzymes or, less likely, an increased synthesis of non-lysosomal acid phosphatase and β-glucuronidase.

One method for stabilizing lysosomal membranes has been treatment with hydrocortisone [38]. If the mechanism operating in our experiment was dependent on an increase in lysosomal enzyme mobility, then the hydrocortisone treatment should reduce this mobility. Therefore, cultures were prepared in duplicate with and without hydrocortisone (5μg/ml). At different periods, acid phosphatase and β-glucuronidase activities were determined. The results showed that the activity of these enzymes as assayed in crude homogenates increased with aging in the presence or absence of hydrocortisone. In addition, the subcellular distribution of acid phosphatase and β-glucuronidase was not affected by the hydrocortisone treatment. The presence of hydrocortisone, however, produced a striking prolongation of the life span of WI-38 cells. In a series of experiments in which cultures were carried in duplicate, with and without hydrocortisone (5 μg/ml), from passage levels in the very early 20's to the end of the life span, the highest passages attained in the presence and absence of hydrocortisone, respectively, were 66 vs 54, 52 vs 43, and 54 vs 45.

A similar extension of the life span of diploid human
cells with cortisone has been reported by Macieira-
Coelho [39]. On the basis of actual cell numbers, as
well as the number of subcultivations, this extension
of life span in WI-38 cells was a real phenomenon and not
an artifact. Figure 5 shows the results of one of these
experiments. For this study, cells were subcultured at
a ratio of 1:4 (2 doublings = 2 passages) each week. As
the cells approached the end of their life span, the
amount of time necessary to achieve confluency became
extended, and the cells were fed with fresh medium each
week, but subcultivated only when they had reached confluency. When more than one week was required to attain
confluency, the next subcultivation was made at a 1:2
ratio (1 doubling = 1 passage). The points in Figure 5
where the arrows cross the abscissa indicate the passage
level at which the cells, after continual refeedings with
fresh medium, were nevertheless unable to proliferate and
achieve confluency.

Figure 6 summarizes the results of a number of other
experiments in which hydrocortisone was added or removed
at different points in the life cycle. In the absence of
hydrocortisone (bar 1, top of figure) the life span was
45 passages. Addition of hydrocortisone at passage 44
had no recovery effect on sister cultures (bar 2). Addition of hydrocortisone at passages 29 and 39, however,
did extend the life span approximately 9-10%. Hydrocortisone added at passage 21 extended the life span
about 20%. It is possible that the overall life span
would be greatly extended if hydrocortisone was included
in the media of primary explants.

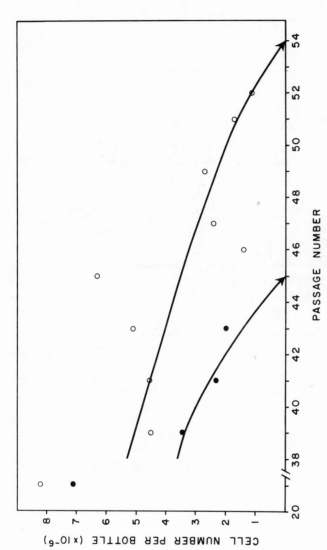

Fig. 5. The effect of hydrocortisone on the life span of WI-38 cells. The points where the arrows cross the abscissa indicate the passage levels at which the cells were no longer able to achieve confluency. ●, control; O, hydrocortisone, 5 μg/ml.

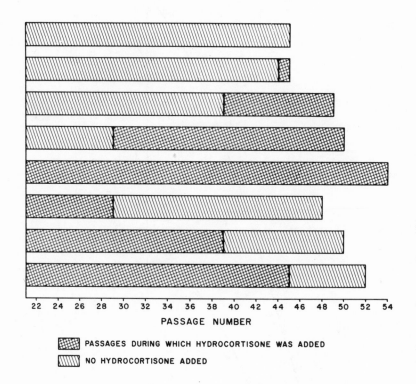

Fig. 6. The effect of the addition and removal of hydrocortisone on the life span of WI-38 cells.

The remaining three bars on the graph show the reverse experiment. Three other sister cultures were cultivated in the presence of hydrocortisone beginning with passage 21, and the hydrocortisone was removed at passages 29, 39, and 45. Again, there seems to be a direct relationship between the number of passages during which the cells were maintained on hydrocortisone and the eventual life span of the culture.

This effect may be much more complicated than simply stablization of the lysosomal enzymes. An alternative explanation for the hydrocortisone effect can be based on reports involving several cell culture systems in which the addition of hydrocortisone to the medium induces the formation of specific proteins, for example, alkaline phosphatase [40] and tyrosine transaminase [41, 42]. More recently, it has been demonstrated that the addition of hydrocortisone to chick embryo retinal cells induces the premature synthesis of the enzyme glutamine synthetase. This induction requires the synthesis of specific messenger RNA and its subsequent translation in order to make the specific enzyme protein [43].

Similarly, we have observed what may be induction of alkaline phosphatase in WI-38 cells grown in the presence of hydrocortisone [44]. The relationship between the induction of alkaline phosphatase and the increase in the life span of WI-38 cells is obscure. However, a consideration of the general phenomenon of hydrocortisone-induced protein synthesis may suggest a mechanism by which the hormone increases the longevity of WI-38 cells.

Following each division of WI-38 cells a certain percentage of the daughter cells in the population may be
committed to becoming non-dividers, i.e., they may lose
their ability to proliferate. This percentage of non-
dividers would increase with each passage number, thus
accounting for the phase III phenomenon and the eventual
degeneration of the culture. We might postulate that
the mechanism by which a cell becomes a non-divider involves the loss of the ability to synthesize a protein
necessary for the initiation of the division cycle. In
WI-38 cells hydrocortisone can presumably induce the
synthesis of this protein. Griffin and Ber [45] have
shown that alkaline phosphatase induction by hydrocortisone in synchronized cultures of HeLa cells occurs ex-
clusively in the synthetic (S) phase of the cell cycle.
Only at this stage can the appropriate messenger RNA be
synthesized. If this same mechanism also operates for
our hypothetical division-initiating protein, then the
effectiveness of hydrocortisone in WI-38 cultures would
be limited to cells in the S phase. Cells in G2 phase,
or mitosis, would have to complete the division cycle and
fulfill their commitment to become dividers or non-dividers.
Dividers would pass through G1, enter S phase and be re-
scued from producing non-dividing daughters by the action
of hydrocortisone. Assuming that this message is relatively short-lived and does not survive mitosis, then the
addition of hydrocortisone at the end of the life span of
the cells (Figure 6) would have no rescue effect since
most of the cells are blocked in the G1 or G2 phase [24].
In the more actively proliferating early passage cultures,
the probability of finding cells in S phase is higher than
in late passage cultures since the percentage of non-
dividers is smaller. Thus, the earlier in the population

life history hydrocortisone is added, the longer the extension of the life span. Finally, the culture will eventually degenerate despite the presence of hydro-cortisone, since the probability of finding cells in S phase will decrease with increasing passages or sub-cultivations.

SUMMARY AND CONCLUSION

In summary, we can say that: 1) Energy metabolism appears to proceed unchanged during aging in culture. 2) Transketolase and 6-phosphogluconate dehydrogenase show age-associated decreases in activity in WI-38 cells, while transaldolase and 6-phosphogluconate dehydrogenase activities are reduced in transformed cells as compared with actively proliferating WI-38 cells. 3) Senescent cells are incapable of division, probably because of an inability to initiate the synthesis of DNA (as suggested by the work of Macieira-Coelho and our measurements). 4) The RNA content of aging cells is disproportionately increased. 5) Cell growth continues in the absence of cell division, resulting in an increased size of the cells. 6) The specific activity of lysosomal enzymes is increased during aging. 7) Hydrocortisone or cortisone extends the life span of the cell.

Our working hypothesis at present is that some pro-tein with either enzymatic or structural activity which is necessary for the initiation of DNA synthesis cannot be produced. This could be the result of a transcrip-tional or translational mishap, either accidental or pro-grammed.

The cell can then no longer divide, but it can continue to grow and actively metabolize. The disproportionate increase in RNA may reflect a compensatory reaction of some sort and the resulting unbalanced growth
could trigger activation of the lysosomal enzymes and cause
cell death. Hydrocortisone presumably has a multiple effect,
being involved in the stabilization of the lysosomal membranes and more importantly in the induction of proteins
necessary for continued cell proliferation.

ACKNOWLEDGMENTS

The author is grateful to Dr. David Kritchevsky for
helpful suggestions and discussions and to Joan Kabakjian,
Susan Godfrey, Carol Gianniti, Pauline Sallata, and
Allen Opalek for their expert technical assistance in
various phases of this work.

REFERENCES

1. L. Hayflick and P.S. Moorhead, "The serial cultivation
   of human diploid cell strains," Exp. Cell Res.,
   25:585, 1961.
2. L. Hayflick, "The limited in vitro lifetime of human
   diploid cell strains," Exp. Cell Res., 37:614, 1965.
3. A.J. Girardi, F.C. Jensen, and H. Koprowski, "SV40
   transformation of human diploid cells: Crisis and recovery," J. Cell. Comp. Physiol., 65:69, 1965.
4. V.J. Cristofalo and D. Kritchevsky, "Growth and glycolysis in the human diploid cell strain WI-38," Proc.
   Soc. Exp. Biol. Med., 118:1109, 1965.
5. P.F. Kruse, Jr., and E. Miedema, "Glucose uptake related to proliferation of animal cells in vitro," Proc.
   Soc. Exp. Biol. Med., 119:1110, 1965.

6. V.J. Cristofalo and D. Kritchevsky, "Respiration and glycolysis in the human diploid cell strain WI-38," J. Cell. Comp. Physiol., 67:125, 1965.

7. H. Eagle, "The minimum vitamin requirements of the L and HeLa cells in tissue culture, the production of specific vitamin deficiencies and their cure," J. Exp. Med., 102:595, 1955.

8. W.W. Umbreit, R.H. Burris, and J.F. Stauffer, Manometric Techniques, Minneapolis, Minn., Burgess, 1957.

9. C.E. Shonk and G.E. Boxer, "Enzyme patterns in human tissues. I. Methods for the determination of glycolytic enzymes," Cancer Res. 24:709, 1964.

10. F. Novello and P. McLean, "The pentose phosphate pathway of glucose metabolism. Measurement of the non-oxidative reactions of the cycle," Biochem. J., 107:775, 1968.

11. G. Ashwell and J. Hickman, "Enzymatic formation of xylulose 5-phosphate from ribose 5-phosphate in spleen," J. Biol. Chem., 226:65, 1957.

12. O.H. Lowry, N.J. Rosebrough, A.L. Farr and R.J. Randall, "Protein measurement with the Folin phenol reagent," J. Biol. Chem. 193:265, 1951.

13. N. Hakami and D.A. Pious, "Mitochondrial enzyme activity in "senescent" and virus-transformed human fibroblasts," Exp. Cell. Res. 53:135, 1968.

14. J.M. Reiner, "The effect of age on the carbohydrate metabolism of tissue homogenates," J. Gerontol., 2:315, 1947.

15. H.A. Rafsky, B. Newman and A. Horonick, "Age differences in respiration of guinea pig tissue," J. Gerontol., 7:38, 1952.

16. C.H. Barrows, Jr., M.J. Yiengst and N.W. Shock,
    "Senescence and the metabolism of various tissues
    of rats," J. Gerontol., 13:351, 1958.
17. P.H. Gold, M.V. Gee and B.L. Strehler, "Effect of
    age on oxidative phosphorylation in the rat," J.
    Gerontol., 23:509, 1968.
18. C.W. Parr, "Inhibition of phosphoglucose isomerase,"
    Nature, 178:1401, 1956.
19. E. Miedema and P.F. Kruse, Jr., "Enzyme activities
    and protein contents of animal cells cultured under
    perfusion conditions," Biochem. Biophys. Res. Comm.,
    20:528, 1965.
20. E. Noltmann and F.H. Bruns, "Reindarstellung und
    Eigenschaften von Phosphoglucose-isomerase aus
    Hefe," Biochem. Z. 331:436, 1959.
21. E. Volkin and W.E. Cohn, "Estimation of nucleic
    acids," in: D. Glick, Ed., Methods of Biochemical
    Analysis, New York, Interscience Publishers, 1954,
    p. 287.
22. G.T. Rudkin, D.A. Hungerford and P.C. Nowell, "DNA
    content of chromosome Ph[1] and chromosome 21 in human
    chronic granulocytic leukemia," Science, 144:1229,
    1964.
23. T.A. Tedesco and W.J. Mellman, "Desoxyribonucleic
    acid assay as a measure of cell number in preparations
    from monolayer cell cultures and blood leucocytes,"
    Exp. Cell Res., 45:230, 1967.
24. A. Macieira-Coelho, J. Pontén and L. Philipson,
    "The division cycle and RNA-synthesis in diploid
    human cells at different passage levels in vitro,"
    Exp. Cell Res., 42:673, 1966.

25. J.W.I.M. Simons, "The use of frequency distribution of cell diameters to characterize cell populations in tissue cultures," Exp. Cell Res., 45:336, 1967.

26. V.J. Cristofalo, B.V. Howard and D. Kritchevsky, "Biochemistry of human cells in culture," in: U. Gallo and L. Santamaria, Eds., Research Progress in Organic-Biological and Medicinal Chemistry, Amsterdam, Noord Hollandsche Uitgevers-MIJ, in press.

27. V.J. Wulff, M. Piekielniak, and M.J. Wayner, "The ribonucleic acid (RNA) content of tissues of rats of different ages," J. Gerontol. 18:322, 1963.

28. R. Weber, "Behavior and properties of acid hydrolases in regressing tails of tadpoles during spontaneous and induced metamorphosis in vitro," in: A.V.S. DeReuck and Margaret P. Cameron, Eds., CIBA Found. Symp. on Lysosomes, Boston, Mass., Little, Brown, 1963, p. 282.

29. A.C. Allison and G.R. Paton, "Chromosome damage in human diploid cells following activation of lysosomal enzymes," Nature, 207:1170, 1965.

30. G. Bernardi and C. Sadron, "Studies on acid dexoyribonuclease I. Kinetics of the initial degradation of deoxyribonucleic acid by acid deoxyribonuclease," Biochem., 3:1411, 1964.

31. O.A. Bessey, O.H. Lowry, M.J. Brock, "A method for the rapid determination of alkaline phosphatase with five cubic millimeters of serum," J. Biol. Chem., 164:321, 1946.

32. W.H. Fishman, "β-glucuronidase," in: Methods of Enzymatic Analysis, H. Bergmeyer, Ed., New York, Acad. Press, 1963, p. 869.

33. A. Zorzoli, "The influence of age on phosphatase activity in the liver of the mouse," J. Gerontol., 10:156, 1955.

34. P. Gedigk, and E. Bontke, "Über den Nachweis von
    Hydrolytischen Enzymen in Lipopigmenten," Z. Zellforsch.,
    44:495, 1956.

35. E. Essner and A. Novikoff, "Human hepatocelullar pig-
    ments and lysosomes, J. Ultrastruct. Res. 3:374, 1960.

36. G.H. Bourne, "General aspects of aging in cells from
    a physiological point of view," in: B.L. Strehler
    et al., Eds., Biology of Aging, Washington, D.C.,
    Am. Inst. Biol. Sci., 1960, No.6, p. 133.

37. V.J. Cristofalo, J.R. Kabakjian and D. Kritchevsky,
    "Heterogeneity of acid phosphatase in the human dip-
    loid cell strain WI-38." Proc. Soc. Exp. Biol. Med.,
    126:648, 1967.

38. G. Weissman and J. Dingle, "Release of lysosomal
    protease by ultraviolet irradiation and inhibition
    by hydrocortisone," Exp. Cell Res., 25:207, 1961.

39. A. Macieira-Coelho, "Action of cortisone on human
    fibroblasts in vitro," Experientia, 22:390, 1966.

40. R.P. Cox and C.M. MacLeod, "Alkaline phosphatase con-
    tent and the effects of prednisolone on mammalian
    cells in culture," J. Gen. Physiol., 45:439, 1962.

41. H.C. Pitot, C. Peraino, P.A. Morse, and V.R. Potter,
    "Hepatomas in tissue culture compared with adapting
    liver in vivo," Nat.Cancer Inst. Monograph 13:229,
    1964.

42. E.B. Thompson, G.M. Tomkins and J.F. Curran, "In-
    duction of tyrosine α-ketoglutarate transaminase
    by steroid hormones in a newly established tissue
    culture cell line. Proc. Nat. Acad. Sci. U.S.A.,
    56:296, 1966.

43. L. Rief-Lehrer and H. Amos, "Hydrocortisone re-
    quirements for the induction of glutamine synthetase
    in chick-embryo retinas," Biochem. J., 106:425, 1968.
44. V.J. Cristofalo and J. Kabakjian, "In preparation".
45. M.J. Griffin and R. Ber, "Cell cycle events in the
    hydrocortisone regulation of alkaline phosphatase in
    HeLa S$_3$ cells," J. Cell Biol., 40:297, 1969.

THE DECREASED GROWTH POTENTIAL IN VITRO

OF HUMAN FIBROBLASTS OF ADULT ORIGIN[+]

A. MACIEIRA-COELHO

Institut de Cancérologie
et d'Immunogénétique
94-Villejuif, France

The growth declining stage (phase III) of human embryonic fibroblasts (1), is characterized by marked changes in the kinetics of the cell division cycle (2). This is already apparent in the growth curves obtained from daily cell counts performed between the time of subcultivation and the time growth stops (2). The growth curves show that phase III cells have a longer lag phase (time between inoculum and the first net increase in the population), a shorter period of active growth and a saturation density which is considerably less than the one found in early passage cultures (phase II). These changes in growth are due to a longer generation time caused by a prolongation of the G_1 and G_2 periods of the cell cycle, to a decrease in the amount of cells engaged in the division cycle and to an increase of the nondividing population between subcultivation and the time growth stops.

Hayflick (3) found that human fibroblastic cultures of adult origin have a shorter lifespan in vitro than human embryonic fibroblasts. This seems to show that adult cells have a decreased doubling potential as compared with embryonic

---

[+] Part of the data presented is reproduced with the permission of the Rockfeller University Press.

cells and is in favor of the concept of aging at a cellular level to explain the growth decline and death of these populations (1).

The present work was performed to see if adult fibroblasts show in early passage the same changes in the kinetics of the cell division cycle as late passage embryonic cells. This in fact, seems to be the case.

MATERIALS AND METHODS

The HEB line of fetal lung origin (4) and the 2S line derived from an adult skin biopsy (5) were used maintained in Eagle's minimal essential medium supplemented with penicillin (100 U/ml), aureomycin or kanamycin (50μg/ml) and 10 % calf serum.

Cell counts and determination of cell size were done with an electronic counter as described (6).

For autoradiography cells were grown in Petri dishes containing coverslips. Tritium labelled thymidine (s.a. 1.9 c/mM) in a final concentration of 0.01μc/ml was added to the cultures for variable periods of time depending on the experiment. Coverslips were removed, washed in PBS and fixed in acetic acid-methanol (1 : 3) for 1 hour and dried. The coverslips were glued to a microscopic glass slide by Canada Balsam, dried, dipped in a gelatine-chrome alum solution and coated with Kodak AR10 film.

After a 7 day exposure the preparations were developed for 4 minutes in Kodak D-19B, kept for 10 minutes in Kodak Acid Fixer and washed for 10 minutes in running tap water. Staining was done immediately afterwards in a 0.05 % (w/v) solution of toluidine blue for 3-5 minutes. Film adhering to the back of the slide was scraped off and after drying the preparations were ready for analysis. One thousand nuclei were observed in the determination of the proportion of labelled interphase nuclei.

RESULTS

Phase II populations of embryonic and of
adult origin were pooled separately and subcultivated into new Petri dishes so that each culture
vessel received 10^6 cells. H^3-TdR was added daily
to duplicate cultures and the cells fixed 24 hours
after receiving the labelled precursor. Duplicate
sister cultures were counted each day until no
mitotic activity was observed. As can be seen in
fig. 1 the maximum amount of cells synthesizing
DNA during a 24 hour period was considerably less
in early passage adult cells than in early passage
embryonic cells. The percentage of cells entering
DNA synthesis each day after subcultivation fluc-
tuated widely in adult populations. Sister cultures labelled continuously from the time of inoculation to the time growth stopped showed that 97 %
of the cells entered DNA synthesis in embryonic
cultures while only 66 % of the cells did it in
adult cultures during that passage. It can also be
seen from the growth curves that adult phase II
cells had a longer lag period and that they took
a longer time to reach the saturation density

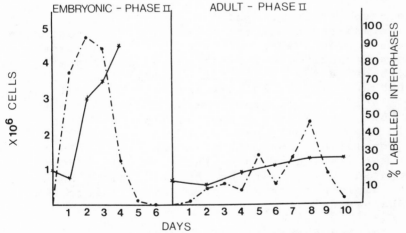

Fig. 1. Cell counts plotted semi-logarith-
mically (x————x) and percentage labelled
interphase plotted arithmetically (·—·—·)
during each 24 hours after subcultivation
in HEB and 2S cultures.

which is obtained at a considerably lower figure
than in embryonic cells. The doubling time measured from the portion of the growth curves during
which a net increase in the population takes place,
is very prolonged in adult populations.

To see if the slow growth of adult cells was
due to a prolongation of the S period, the time
spent in DNA synthesis was measured as described
by Stanners and Till (7). H^3-TdR was added to ex-
ponentially growing cultures. Duplicate samples
were removed at hourly intervals thereafter and
processed for autoradiography. The time interval
between the first appearance of labelled metaphases
and the point when the number of grains over metaphases reaches a plateau during the continuous labelling corresponds to the length of the S period.
For the determination of the number of grains over
metaphases, the grain counts of 100 labelled metaphases at each hour after adding the H^3-TdR were
plotted as histograms. The cumulative percentage
of such labelled metaphases plotted against grain
counts on probability paper gave straight lines
(fig. 2). The intersection of the straight lines
with the 50 % line represents the peak value of
metaphase grain counts. As shown in fig. 3 labelled metaphases are first seen in the embryonic population from the second hour. The time between
the appearance of the first labelled metaphases
and the time the peak grain count reaches a plateau
is 6 hours. In the cultures of cells of adult origin, labelled metaphases are only found from the
5th hour. The S period however lasts the same time
as in the embryonic cell cultures (fig. 3). In both
the populations the peak metaphase grain count reaches the plateau at about the same value (80grains/
metaphase) which is to be expected, since both are
human diploid lines and hence have the same amount
of DNA per cell.

The percentage of labelled metaphases from
the same experiment was plotted against time. As
shown in fig. 4, 100 % of the metaphases are labelled from the 5th hour in embryonic cell cultures.
In adult cell populations however, 100 % labelled
metaphases were never seen within the experimental

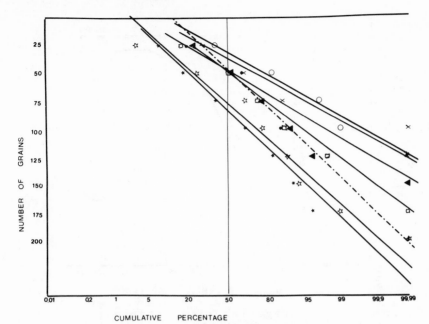

Fig. 2. Cumulative percentage of metaphase grain counts found in 2S cells at each hour after adding the H^3-TdR; plotted on probability paper.

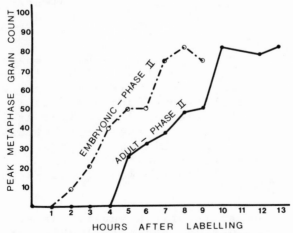

Fig. 3. Peak metaphase grain counts at each hour during a continuous labelling of logarithmically growing HEB (∘—·—∘) and 2 S (•——•) cultures.

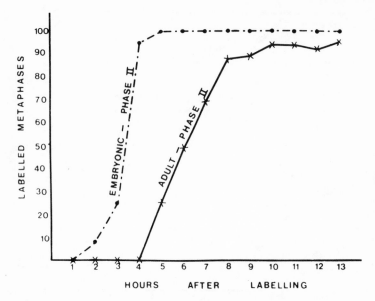

Fig. 4. Percentage labelled metaphases in
the same experiment as the one shown in
fig. 3. HEB (•—·—•) and 2S (x———x) cultures.

time. This shows that in adult cell cultures in
phase II there are cells with a G_2 period of at
least 13 hours.

It has been shown previously by Simons (8)
that human fibroblasts in phase III are larger
than cells in phase II. For this reason we compared the size distribution of phase II and III embryonic cells with phase II adult cells. As is
shown in fig. 5 the mode of the distributions
found in phase II adult cells and in phase III
embryonic cells coincide and are skewed to the
right when compared with the mode found in phase
II embryonic cells.

The line of adult origin entered after 60
passages a final period (phase III) where growth
declined which was followed by cell death.

To see if the increase in cell size could influence the saturation density, phase II and phase

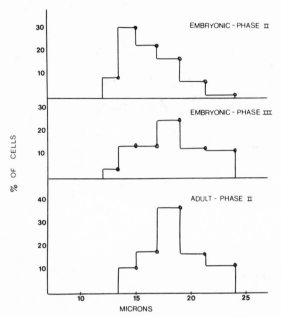

Fig. 5. Distribution of cell diameters
expressed in microns found in phase II
and III HEB and phase II   2S populations.

III HEB cultures were subcultivated into new vessels so that one group received 10^6 phase II cells/
petri dish, another group 4 x 10^5 phase II cells,
a third group 4 x 10^5 phase III cells, a fourth
group 4 x 10^5 phase II and 4 x 10^5 phase III cells
simultaneously in each Petri dish and finally a 5th
group with 4 x 10^5 phase II and 8 x 10^5 phase III
cells in each dish. Cell counts were performed
daily in each group. Growth curves are represented
in fig. 6. As can be seen, the two groups with
phase II cells alone reached the same terminal cell
density despite of the different inocula. The group
with 4 x 10^5 phase II and 4 x 10^5 phase III cells
reached a terminal cell density 18 % lower than the
terminal density of phase II cells grown alone. The
group with 4 x 10^5 and 8 x 10^5 phase III cells combined reached a terminal density 39 % lower than
the density of phase II cells grown alone. Finally
phase III cells grown alone reached a density 57 %
lower than the density of phase II cells also grown

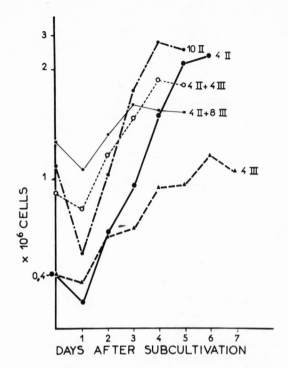

Fig. 6. Growth curves of phase II and III
HEB cells grown separately and cocultivated
after different inocula. For further explanation see text.

alone. To check if the two populations were present in
the mixed cultures, the first day after subcultivation
cells from each group were analysed to determine their
size distribution. Results are presented in fig. 7.
It can be seen that phase II cells have a diameter distribution with a mode between 13.4 and 15.4μ, while phase
III cells have a mode between 16.9 and 19μ. When phase II
and phase III cultures were cocultivated, the groups
showed two peaks: one between 13.4 and 15μ and the other
between 16.9 and 19μ. It is clear from this experiment
that the presence of phase III cells in increased amounts
decreases proportionally the final density reached by the
mixed population.

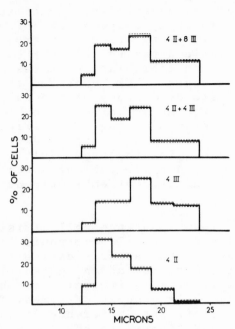

Fig. 7. Size distribution found on the
first day after subcultivation in the
same experiment as the one represented
in fig. 6. The interrupted lines represent the 95 % confidence limits.

DISCUSSION

Even in the early history of tissue culture, it was observed that survival and growth of
cell cultures varied within wide limits. Whereas
some times cultures only multiplied for relatively
short periods, in other instances they had an apparently unlimited capacity for multiplication. Somatic cells were conceived of as potentially immortal
and the failure to divide indefinitely was general-
ly thought to be caused by deficiencies in the
artificial environment.

Human fibroblasts were successively maintained in vitro for long periods of time by Swim et
al. (9), Puck et al. (10), Hsu et al. (11) and by
Hayflick et al. (1). The last investigators

however challenged the accepted view that in vitro
deficiencies were entirely responsible for the failure of indefinite cell propagation in vitro. To
explain the invariable degeneration that eventually
terminated their human fibroblast cultures after a
large number of passages, they suggested the exis-
tence of an intrinsic deficiency of the cells which
only permitted a limited number of cell doublings and
which is the expression of aging at a cellular level (1). This idea was further supported by the
fact that cultures originating from adult human
donors had a decreased cell doubling potential
when compared with cultures of embryonic origin
(3).

Previous studies (2) of the cell division
cycle in phase II and phase III embryonic fibroblasts showed that in the latter, less cells were
capable of entering division at any given time and
that those that initiated their cycle were hetero-
geneous concerning their generation times. Their
seemed to be no significant difference in the time
for DNA synthesis and mitosis in the two populations. The major differences between phase II and
phase III cells which could possibly account for
the prolonged generation time of the latter cells
resided in the G_1 and the G_2 periods. The present
work shows that human fibroblastic cultures origi-
nated from an adult donor show already in early
passages the same pattern of growth which was found
in embryonic cultures during the declining period
that precedes death of the population. This pattern
consists in a wide fluctuation and a decreased number of cells synthesizing DNA during a 24 hour period, a decreased number of cells entering the
division cycle between subcultivation and resting
stage, a lower saturation density, a fraction of
cells delayed in the G_2 period and a longer doubling time.

Since it was shown by Simons (8) that cells
in phase III are larger than cells in phase II,
the size distribution of early passage adult cells
was measured and compared with the one of early
and late passage embryonic cultures. The data shows
that phase II adult cells have a size distribution

identical to phase III embryonic cells. This increase in size could be in part responsible for
the lower saturation density observed in phase III
embryonic and in phase II adult cells. Results seem
to show that the presence of phase III cells in
mixed populations with phase II cells decreases
the saturation density proportionally to the amount
of phase III cells inoculated. This could be due
to a competition for surface area of attachment in
the culture vessel ; phase III cells being larger
need probably a larger area of attachment per cell.

In general cells which divide very little
seem to increase in size. Very large cells are
found in vivo in tissues with a slow rate of division. Thus the increase in size described above
could be a consequence of the slowdown of cell division. If this is the case, the chain of events
could be : decrease in the division rate ⟶
increase in size ⟶ decrease in the saturation
density which aggravates the growth decline.

No explanation has yet been found for the
slow transit (2) of "old" cells through the division cycle. Since the time of DNA synthesis and
mitosis seems to be unimpaired the mechanisms responsible for the slow-down are probably located in
the periods preceding those two events of the cell
cycle.

SUMMARY

The growth of human fibroblasts of adult origin was analysed during the first part of their
life in vitro when proliferation is more active
(phase II). Results show that they present already
in phase II the same growth patterns which were
found to take place when fibroblasts of embryonic
origin reach the declining stage (phase III) of
their in vitro lifetime. Results are in favor of
the idea that adult fibroblasts are "older" than
embryonic fibroblasts. The mechanisms implicated
in the growth decline seem to be localized in the
periods that lead to DNA synthesis and mitosis
rather than in these processes themselves. The
decrease in the saturation density observed in

"aging" cells seems to be due at least in part,
to the increase in cell size.

REFERENCES

1. L. Hayflick and P.M. Moorhead, "The serial cultivation of human diploid cell strains," Exp.
Cell. Res., 25 : 585, 1961.
2. A. Macieira-Coelho, J. Ponten and L. Philipson,
"The division cycle and RNA-synthesis in diploid
human cells at different passage levels in
vitro," Exp. Cell. Res., 42 : 673, 1966.
3. L. Hayflick, "The limited in vitro lifetime of
human diploid cell strains," Exp. Cell. Res.,
37 : 614, 1965.
4. A. Macieira-Coelho, J. Ponten and L. Philipson,
"Inhibition of the division cycle in confluent
cultures of human fibroblasts in vitro," Exp.
Cell. Res., 43 : 20, 1966.
5. J. Ponten and E. Saksela, "Two established in
vitro cell lines from human mesenchymal tu-
mours," Int. J. Cancer 2 : 434, 1967.
6. R.J. Santen, "Automated estimation of diploid
and tetraploid nuclei with an electronic parti-
cle counter", Exp. Cell. Res., 40 : 413, 1965.
7. C.P. Stanners and J.E. Till, "DNA synthesis in
individual L-strain mouse cells," Bioch. Bioph.
Acta 37 : 406, 1960.
8. J.W. Simons, "The use of frequency distributions
of cell diameters to characterize cell populations in tissue culture," Exp. Cell. Res., 45:
336, 1967.
9. H.E. Swim and R.F. Parker, "Culture characteristics of human fibroblasts propagated serially,"
Am. J. Hygiene 66 : 235, 1957.
10. T.T. Puck, S.J. Cieciura and A. Robinson,
"Genetics of somatic mammalian cells. III. Long-
term cultivation of euploid cells from human
and animal subjects," J. Exptl. Med., 108 : 945,
1958.
11. T.C. Hsu and D.S. Kellog Jr., "Primary cultivation and continuous propagation in vitro of
tissues from small biopsy specimen," J. Natl.
Canc. Inst., 25 : 221, 1960.

RNA AND DNA METABOLISM IN AGING CULTURED CELLS

Jiří Michl and Jana Svobodová

Institute of Physiology, Czechoslovak Academy
of Sciences, and the Research Institute for
Medical Use of Radioisotopes, Prague, Czechoslovakia

In contrast to heteroploid cell lines, human diploid cell
lines have a finite lifetime in vitro; the ultimate fate
of human diploid cells growing in vitro has been studied
by Hayflick and Moorhead [1] and by Hayflick [2]. However, biochemical and cytophysiological characterization
of young and old diploid cells, as compared to cells that
can be cultivated indefinitely, has been limited to only
a few studies.

Until very recently, serum proteins were thought to
be essential for the growth of all animal cell types in
vitro; new evidence indicates that serum macromolecules
are not essential for the optimal growth of certain cell
lines. These cell lines, however, have developed as a
result of adaptation or selection; the growth of diploid
cell lines has never been shown to occur in protein-free
medium. On the basis of investigations carried out in our
laboratory in recent years, we have reached the conclusion
that animal cells can be cultivated in synthetic medium
containing growth-promoting α-globulin. The growth-promoting α-globulin of calf serum is a protein complex which
contains both protein and non-protein components [3,4].

The presence of this protein permits the cultivation of
mammalian cells in a synthetic medium, regardless of
whether they are heteroploid or human diploid cell lines
[3,4,5]. In this sense, the growth-promoting α-globulin
is an essential component for non-adapted cells. The present communication describes the relationship between
the soluble pool and metabolic state of RNA and the influence of the growth-promoting α-globulin on RNA and DNA
synthesis in human cells in vitro.

MATERIALS AND METHODS

The diploid cell strain used, LEP 14, was established from human fetal lung tissue [5]; this fibroblast strain, characterized by the properties described
for similar lines by Hayflick and Moorhead [1], could be
subcultured for a limited number of times before it became senescent and died. In accordance with the procedure of Kritchevsky and Howard [6], early and late
passage cells were divided at a passage level which represented seven-tenths of the lifespan. Since heteroploid cell lines have an unlimited growth potential in
vitro, HeLa cells were used for comparison with diploid
cells.

The cells were cultivated in a synthetic medium [7]
supplemented with the growth-promoting α-globulin, or
with calf serum, and after labeling with ^{32}P or ^3H-uri-
dine the radioactivity of the TCA-soluble and TCA-in-
soluble compounds, as well as RNA, DNA and residual protein, was determined. Carbamyl phosphate-aspartate transcarbamylase (ATCase) was assayed by the method of Koritz
and Cohen [8] using a modification described by Consigli

and Ginsberg [9].

The growth-promoting α-globulin contains phosphate groups, probably in the form of carbamyl phosphate [10]. For this reason we tried to ascertain whether the ^{32}P-labeled protein was utilized by the cells. The growth-promoting α-globulin (2 g in 100 ml water) was exposed to $Na_2H^{32}PO_4$ (2 mC) for 24 hr at 4°C and after incubation, the solution was dialyzed. The synthetic medium, containing, in addition to the defined components, unlabeled calf serum albumin (0.1%), was supplemented with ^{32}P-labeled or unlabeled α-globulin (0.2 mg per ml of medium). Control medium, containing unlabeled α-globulin , was supplemented immediately before use with $Na_2H^{32}PO_4$; both media contained equal amounts of radioactivity.

In preliminary experiments the ^{32}P pools in HeLa cells and in human diploid cells in the middle and late passages were compared. The levels of ^{32}P intermediates were different in HeLa cells and in young diploid cells; furthermore, old diploid cells had a much larger pool than young cells (Table I).

RESULTS AND DISCUSSION

From the results it was assumed that a greater turnover of macromolecular cell components, containing ^{32}P (predominantly RNA) rather than an increased entrance of ^{32}P into the old cells was responsible for the increase of radioactivity in the cell water. At the same time,

Table I. The ^{32}P Pool Formed in HeLa Cells and
in Human Diploid Cells during a Short-term Cultivation (5 hr, 37°C, 0.1μC of $Na_2H^{32}PO_4$ per ml of
synthetic medium supplemented with 10% calf serum).

^{32}P POOL

CELLS	% OF RADIOACTIVITY IN CELL WATER MEDIUM = 100 %
HELA	470
LEP 14 - 15th PASSAGE	286
LEP 14 - 36th PASSAGE	516

it is possible that the incorporation of TCA-soluble ^{32}P
into RNA and DNA decreased in old diploid cells.

To verify our hypothesis, the stability of RNA, which
is the most important macromolecular compound able to be
in equilibrium with ^{32}P acid-soluble compounds, was
studied in HeLa cells and in human diploid cells. For
these studies, the cells were cultivated for 18 hr in
serum-supplemented medium containing ^{3}H-uridine. After
this period, the cultures were washed and the synthetic
medium, without serum or ^{3}H-uridine, was added to one-half
of the cultures. After an additional 48 hr at 37°C, the

Table II. The Amounts of ³H-uridine-containing Compounds in HeLa Cells and in Human Diploid Cells (The cells were incubated in serum-supplemented medium containing 1.0 µC per ml of ³H-uridine for 18 hr; half of the cultures were incubated for an additional 48 hr in serum-free medium without ³H-uridine).

³H-URIDINE

CELLS	RADIOACTIVITY OF 0.1ml PACKED CELLS c.p.m.				RADIOACTIVITY OF EXPERIMENTAL CELLS % OF CONTROL CELLS	
	CONTROL CELLS		CELLS AFTER THE INCUBATION IN THE SERUM-FREE MEDIUM			
	SOLUBLE POOL	RNA	SOLUBLE POOL	RNA	SOLUBLE POOL	RNA
HELA	130 614	577 491	21 735	550 407	16.6	95.3
LEP 14-16th passage	230 601	343 882	50 327	239 691	21.8	69.7
LEP 14-36th passage	235 502	968 226	32 262	539 078	13.6	55.6

radioactivity in this group of cultures was compared
with control cultures incubated for only 18 hr in the
presence of serum. As shown in Table II, after 48 hr
95.3% of the radioactivity remained in the RNA of HeLa
cells, but only 69.7 and 55.6% in the RNA of young and
old diploid cells.

The reduced breakdown of RNA in HeLa cells was found
to be correlated with the activity of the enzyme
carbamyl phosphate-aspartate transcarbamylase. In HeLa
cells the activity of transcarbamylase was about 200%
of that found in young diploid cells and more than 330%
of that found in old diploid cells (Table III).

Table III. Activity of Carbamyl Phosphate-asparatate
Transcarbamylase in Human Cells Grown in Culture
(Enzyme activity is expressed as micromoles x 10^{-8}
of ureidosuccinate synthetized during one hr incubation at 37°C by enzyme extracted from one cell).

CELLS	UREIDOSUCCINIC ACID FORMED PER CELL PER HOUR / $\mu M \times 10^{-8}$ /
HELA	6.1
L	6.5
LEP 14 - 22nd PASSAGE	3.0
LEP 14 - 41st PASSAGE	1.8

Our data are in accord with results previously reported by Kim and Cohen [11]. The level of transcarbamylase activity has been found to increase during regeneration with the highest activity found in the youngest
fetal livers, decreasing to low levels during development and in the adult animal. Furthermore, a relatively
high level of transcarbamylase activity was demonstrated
in tumour cells. At the same time it is very interesting
to note that our results with human diploid cell cultures,
old and young, are in accordance with the experiments of
Samis, Wulff and Falzone [12] in which they showed a
greater RNA turnover in the nuclei of rat liver cells of
old animals.

Nilausen and Green [13] reported that the cultures
of an established line of mouse fibroblasts (3T3) were
very susceptible to contact inhibition of cell division
and became arrested at confluence. Cells in this stage
were not nutritionally limited and resumed cell division
when a macromolecular substance(s) present in dialyzed
serum was added to temporarily diminish contact inhibition. When cell divisions were induced in this way there
occurred, within 15 min, a rapid increase in the rate of
RNA synthesis; this was followed within 2 hr by an increase in the rate of protein synthesis and many hours
later by the initiation of DNA synthesis and cell division [14]. These results show that stationary phase cells
have sufficient enzymatic machinery to support the rate of
RNA synthesis characteristic of growing cells; the stimu-
lation effected by the serum factor must therefore operate
by increasing the activity of RNA polymerase already present, perhaps by making the DNA template more available
to it [15]. If serum protein(s) is actually involved in

the regulation of RNA synthesis, then one would expect
to see an increase in the utilization of RNA intermediates
and in the stabilization of RNA under the influence of
specific serum protein. Our present experiments on the
influence of serum proteins in cell culture confirm this
prediction. The data in Figure 1 show that the level
of ^{32}P in the TCA-soluble pool is lower in a medium supplemented with calf serum. It is clear from the present
experiments that ^{32}P-intermediates are not incorporated
into RNA and DNA in serum-free medium and that they may
be lost from the cell.

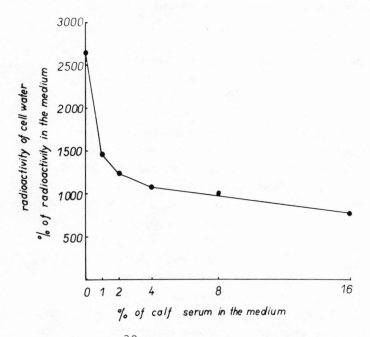

Fig. 1. The ^{32}P pool formed in HeLa cells
incubated in a synthetic medium supplemented
with different amounts of calf serum (18 hr,
37°C, 0.1 μC of $Na_2H^{32}PO_4$ per ml of medium).

The radioactivity is actually lost at a slower rate in medium supplemented with serum than in the absence of serum; this difference can be eliminated by the addition of the growth-promoting α-globulin (Fig. 2).

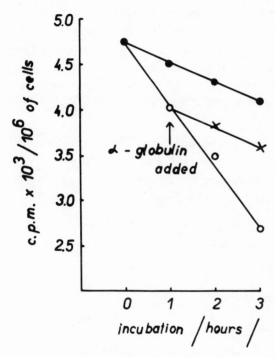

Fig. 2. Loss of radioactivity from ^{32}P-labeled HeLa cells (1 hr, 37°C, 0.1 μC of $Na_2H^{32}PO_4$ per ml of medium). o——o Serum-supplemented medium. x——x Synthetoc medium supplemented with the growth-promoting α-globulin. o——o Synthetic medium.

Thus in serum-free medium, ^{32}P-intermediates are re-
leased from the cells, and biosynthetic and catabolic processes are at first equal; subsequently the degradation
of RNA becomes greater than its biosynthesis and the cells
die. The fact that young diploid cells were able to proliferate in the same pool of medium containing growth-
promoting α-globulin in which older cells were entering
the degenerative phase, does not preclude the possibility
that the utilization of the growth-promoting α-globulin or
some other essential components bound to protein was impaired in the senescent diploid cells.

Table IV. ^{32}P Incorporation into Human Diploid
Cells Incubated in a Synthetic Medium Supplemented with ^{32}P-labeled α-Globulin and a Mixture
of Unlabeled α-Globulin and $Na_2H^{32}PO_4$ (3 hr, 37°C).

	^{32}P-α-GLOBULIN	α-GLOBULIN + $^{32}P_i$
POPULATION DENSITY	50 000 cells/cm^2	
TOTAL RADIOACTIVITY (c.p.m. /10^{6}cells)	3 249	2 508
TCA EXTRACT	74.9 ± 1.1 %	84.7 ± 1.0 %
LIPIDIC EXTRACT	13.6 ± 1.2 %	13.4 ± 0.5 %
RNA	10.2 ± 0.6 %	1.9 ± 0.5 %
DNA	0.8 ± 0.3 %	0.14 ± 0.04 %
PROTEIN	0.1 ± 0.07 %	0.01 ± 0.007 %

The primary function of the growth-promoting
α-globulin in cell culture is still not clear; for this
reason we attempted to verify whether the ^{32}P-labeled
group of the growth-promoting α-globulin was incorporated
in significant amounts into the cells. Data presented
in Table IV demonstrates the distribution of ^{32}P in the
acid-soluble, acid-insoluble, RNA, DNA, and protein
fractions in human diploid cells, incubated 3 hr at 37°C.
As can be seen from Table IV, the distribution of ^{32}P
differed markedly in diploid cells incubated in the presence of labeled α-globulin and in the presence of a
mixture of unlabeled α-globulin and $Na_2H^{32}PO_4$. The differences in RNA and DNA fractions are significant and
most important; they indicate that the growth-promoting
α-globulin can serve as a source of utilizable high-
energy phosphate groups or as a suitable phosphate
carrier.

Kleinsmith, Allfrey and Mirsky [16,17] have presented evidence that phosphoproteins play a role in the
modulation of DNA template activity; they have shown
that phosphorylation of acid extractable proteins in the
nuclear fraction is an energy-linked process. The discovery that phosphoproteins are localized and actively
metabolized in cell nuclei has led to speculations on
the possible role of these proteins in nuclear function.

Human lymphocytes treated with phytohaemagglutinin
undergo extensive template activation, as evidenced by
increased synthesis of RNA. It is clear that the rate
of ^{32}P uptake into nuclear proteins increases in phyto-
haemagglutinin-treated cells. Since ATP is known to be

the immediate phosphate donor, an increased specific
activity of the ATP pool could explain the protein
phosphorylation. However, the increase observed in the
specific activity of the ATP pool was not sufficient to
account for the increase in specific activity of the
phosphoprotein fraction. Kleinsmith, Allfrey and Mirsky
[16] pointed out that the increase in specific activity
of the phosphoprotein fraction can be explained only
in terms of an increased specific activity of the ATP
pool. This does not exclude the possibility that in
these experiments, protein phosphorylation was also influenced by the presence of the growth-promoting α-
globulin in serum-supplemented medium.

                        SUMMARY AND CONCLUSIONS

    Our studies have led to the following conclusions:
Human diploid cells have highly unstable RNA; the ratio
between biosynthesis and degradation of RNA may be the
main factor determining cell vitality in vitro. The
level of ^{32}P in the soluble pool is highest in old cells
and the rate of its uptake and re-utilization into RNA and
DNA decreases so that the amounts of synthesized and de-
graded RNA equilibrate; cell replication stops in these
cells. Growth-promoting α-globulin labeled with ^{32}P
could serve as a source of phosphate groups for RNA and
DNA. Young diploid cells were able to proliferate in the
same pool of medium supplemented with the growth-promoting
α-globulin in which older cells were entering the degenerate phase. It is also possible that the utilization

of some essential component(s) bound to protein became impaired in senescent diploid cells. TCA-soluble
intermediates cannot be re-utilized, biosynthetic and
catabolic processes, which were equal at first, subsequently become unbalanced due to the fact that the degradation of RNA exceeds its biosynthesis, and the cells
then die.

REFERENCES

1. L. Hayflick and P.S. Moorhead, "The serial cultivation
   of human diploid cell strains," Exp. Cell Res.,
   25:585, 1961.
2. L. Hayflick, "The limited in vitro lifetime of human
   diploid cell strains," Exp. Cell Res., 37:614, 1965.
3. J. Michl, "Metabolism of cells in tissue culture
   in vitro. I. The influence of serum protein fractions
   on the growth of normal and neoplastic cells,"
   Exp. Cell Res., 23:324, 1961.
4. J. Michl, "Metabolism of cells in tissue culture
   in vitro. II. Long-term cultivation of cell strains
   and cells isolated directly from animals in a stationary culture," Exp. Cell Res., 26:129, 1962.
5. M. Macek and J. Michl, "Příspěvek ke kultivaci
   lidských diploidních buněk," Acta Univ. Carol. Med.,
   10:519, 1964.
6. D. Kritchevsky and B.V. Howard, "The lipids of human
   diploid cell strain WI-38," Ann. Med. Exp. Fenn.,
   44:343, 1966.
7. J. Michl, "Separation of a low molecular weight factor promoting growth of animal cells in vitro," Folia
   Biol.(Prague), 11:285, 1965.

8. S.B. Koritz and P.P. Cohen, "Colorimetric determination of carbamylamino acids and related compounds,"
J. Biol. Chem., 209:145, 1954.

9. R.A. Consigli and H.S. Ginsberg, "Activity of as-
partate transcarbamylase in uninfected and type 5
adenovirus-infected HeLa cells," J. Bact., 87:1034, 1964.

10. J. Michl, "Carbamyl phosphate as an essential component of the flattening factor for cells in culture,"
Nature, 207:412, 1965.

11. S. Kim and P.P. Cohen, "Transcarbamylase activity in
fetal liver and in liver of partially hepatectomized
parabiotic rats," Arch. Biochem. Biophys., 109:421, 1965.

12. H.V. Samis, V.J. Wulff, and J.A. Falzone, "The incorporation of ^{3}H-cytidine into ribonucleic acid of
liver nuclei of young and old rats," Biochim. Biophys.
Acta, 91:223, 1964.

13. K. Nilausen and H. Green, "Reversible arrest of growth
in Gl of an established fibroblast line (3T3),"
Exp. Cell Res., 40:166, 1965.

14. G.J. Todaro, G.K. Lazar, and H. Green, "The initiation
of cell division in a contact-inhibited mammalian cell
line," J. Cell. Comp. Physiol., 66:325, 1965.

15. S. Bloom, G.J. Todaro, and H. Green, "RNA synthesis
during preparation for growth in a resting population
of mammalian cells," Biochem. Biophys. Res. Comm.,
24:412, 1966.

16. L.J. Kleinsmith, V.G. Allfrey, and A.E. Mirsky, "Phosphoprotein metabolism in isolated lymphocyte nuclei,"
Proc. Nat. Acad. Sci., U.S., 55:1182, 1966.

17. L.J. Kleinsmith, V.G. Allfrey, and A.E. Mirsky, "Phosphorylation of nuclear protein early in the course of
gene activation in lymphocytes," Science, 154:780, 1966.

CELL DEATH IN TISSUE CULTURE

Ivan Stanek

Institute of Histology and Embryology,
Medical Faculty, Komenský University,
Bratislava, Czechoslovakia

Using time-lapse microcinemaphotography, the changes accompanying the degeneration and death of cultures of free phagocytizing cells (granulocytes and marcophages) from embryonic chick spleen and brain were studied.

If the cultures were not transferred to fresh medium within a certain time, degenerative changes began which led ultimately to the disintegration of the tissue components. This degenerative process could be reversed to some extent and was caused by unsuitable, depleted environmental conditions, such as inadequate nutrition, lack of oxygen, and an increasing concentration of toxic metabolic products. Of course, this cellular degeneration and death might also have been caused by pathologic influences. Degeneration occurred both in attached and free-floating cells (the macrophages) in older cultures.

In cultures from nervous tissue, after five or more days without replenishment of the medium, the most notice-

able indication of degeneration was the accumulation
of lipids. The free elements accumulated lipid first,
becoming rounder and more cumbersome in appearance.
Their undulating membranes became less spread out and
the surface activity gradually decreased until the cells
finally became motionless. Disintegration and total
decomposition of the cell then followed. The degeneration of attached cells was often combined with the
sudden tearing apart of the intercellular processes.
The cell then became rounded and disintegrated.

The disintegration of cells which had been treated
with fixatives was essentially a different process. For
example, when formol solution was added to the culture
medium, all the cells became immobile after a very short
time. Thus the fixative caused rapid coagulation which
preserved the appearance of the living cells. (Of
course, structural changes occur in even the finest tissue preparation; for example, the undulating membranes
and fine protoplasmic processes often take on a wrinkled
and ruffled configuration.)

A similar, but less rapid effect was caused by
some of the cytostatic compounds, for example, 6-
azauracil riboside. The first manifestation of the
action of this compound is a reduction in the activity
of the macrophages, gradually leading to total immobilization of the cells. After a certain period of time,
bubble-like cytoplasmic projections emerged from the
motionless cells, and could then separate from the cell
body. Similar changes occurred in attached cells at the
zone of out-growth of the explant.

The death of individual free cells was quite different; no morphologically detectable changes in structure or behavior preceded their death. The free cells behaved normally until they suddenly began to pulsate rapidly in the outer layer of the cytoplasm. Then sudden immobilization occurred. Immediately the neighboring macrophages approached the dead cell, and effected its disintegration and the phagocytosis of its elements. This process was not preceded by any morphologically apparent changes in either the overall appearance of the culture or the appearance of the individual cells.

In our opinion, this process is the manifestation of the death of an individual cell, a physiological process occurring at the end of the lifetime of each cell and unrelated to the process in any other cell.

AUTHOR INDEX

(Underscored numbers indicate complete papers in this volume)

SUBJECT INDEX